# Dementia as Social Experience

A diagnosis of dementia changes the ways people engage with each other – for those living with dementia, as well their families, caregivers, friends, health professionals, neighbours, shopkeepers and the community. Medical understandings, necessary as they are, provide no insights into how we may all live good lives with dementia.

This innovative volume brings together an interdisciplinary group of researchers and practitioners to focus on dementia as lived experience. It foregrounds dementia's social, moral, political and economic dimensions, investigating the challenges of reframing the dementia experience for all involved. Part I critiques the stigmas, the negativity, language and fears often associated with a dementia diagnosis, challenging debilitating representations and examining ways to tackle these. Part II examines proactive practices that can support better long-term outcomes for those living with dementia. Part III looks at the relational aspects of dementia care, acknowledging and going beyond the notion of person-centred care. Collectively, these contributions highlight the social and relational change required to enhance life for those with dementia and those who care for them.

Engaging in a critical conversation around personhood and social value, this book examines the wider social contexts within which dementia care takes place. It calls for social change, and looks for inspiration to the growing movement for relational care and the caring society. *Dementia as Social Experience* is important reading for all those people who, in various ways, are living with dementia, as well as for those working in this area as clinicians, researcher and carers.

**Gaynor Macdonald** is a Social Anthropologist at the University of Sydney, Australia.

**Jane Mears** is Associate Professor of Social Policy at Western Sydney University, Australia.

# Routledge Studies in the Sociology of Health and Illness

**Financing Healthcare in China**
Towards Universal Health Insurance
*Sabrina Ching Yuen Luk*

**Socio-economics of Personalized Medicine in Asia**
*Shirley Hsiao-Li Sun*

**Fathering Children with Autism**
Needs, Practices and Service Use
*Carol Potter*

**Recovery, Mental Health and Inequality**
Chinese Ethnic Minorities as Mental Health Service Users
*Lynn Tang*

**Fertility, Health and Lone Parenting**
European Contexts
*Edited by Fabienne Portier-Le Cocq*

**Transnationalising Reproduction**
Third Party Conception in a Globalised World
*Edited by Róisín Ryan Flood and Jenny Gunnarsson Payne*

**Public Health, Personal Health and Pills**
Drug Entanglements and Pharmaceuticalised Governance
*Kevin Dew*

**Dementia as Social Experience**
Valuing Life and Care
*Edited by Gaynor Macdonald and Jane Mears*

www.routledge.com/Routledge-Studies-in-the-Sociology-of-Health-and-Illness/book-series/RSSHI

# Dementia as Social Experience

Valuing Life and Care

**Edited by Gaynor Macdonald
and Jane Mears**

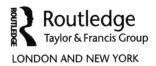

Routledge
Taylor & Francis Group

LONDON AND NEW YORK

First published 2019 by Routledge

2 Park Square, Milton Park, Abingdon, Oxfordshire OX14 4RN
52 Vanderbilt Avenue, New York, NY 10017

*Routledge is an imprint of the Taylor & Francis Group, an informa business*

First issued in paperback 2019

*British Library Cataloguing-in-Publication Data*
A catalogue record for this book is available from the British Library

*Library of Congress Cataloging-in-Publication Data*
A catalog record for this book has been requested

ISBN: 978-0-8153-7457-2 (hbk)
ISBN: 978-0-367-90264-3 (pbk)

Typeset in Times New Roman
by Wearset Ltd, Boldon, Tyne and Wear

# Contents

# Tables

# Contributors

**Meera Agar** works at the University of Technology, Sydney, Australia, is Professor of Palliative Medicine at University of New South Wales, Australia and is a research project lead and chair of the advisory committee at HammondCare.

**Ingrid Amgarth-Duff** is a Research Assistant based at the University of Technology, Sydney, Australia.

**Kirsten Auret** is an Associate Professor at the Rural Clinical School of Western Australia, and a General Physician with speciality training in palliative care. Her research interests include advance care planning, medical education and palliative care.

**Susanne E. Becker** is an early career academic at the Wicking Dementia Research and Education Centre in Hobart, Tasmania. She teaches directly into the online Bachelor of Dementia Care and incorporates her research interests into unit content. She is also evaluating the impact of the Bachelor of Dementia Care as students translate their knowledge into practice. A registered nurse by background, she has worked in the acute, aged care and rural and remote settings from direct nursing care to leadership and management roles.

**Simon Biggs** is Professor of Gerontology and Social Policy, University of Melbourne, Australia, School of Social and Political Sciences/the Brotherhood of Saint Laurence. As an Executive member of the Cognitive Decline Partnership Centre he leads two research projects: public perceptions of dementia and the role of regulation in dementia care. His research interests include intergenerational relations, the ageing life course and public policy.

**Aidan Bindoff** is the statistician for the Wicking Dementia Research and Education Centre, Tasmania. He plays an important role in the statistical evaluation of data, both from students' reflective comments through to laboratory experiments, to help document the role of the Wicking Centre in addressing the cause, care and prevention of dementia.

**Meredith Blake** is an Associate Professor at the University of Western Australia Law School who has published books and articles in the areas of criminal and health law. Her research particularly focuses on advance care planning, end-of-life decision-making, constructing criminal liability and elder law.

**Romola S. Bucks** is a Professor at the University of Western Australia School of Psychological Science, with research interests in ageing, Parkinson's disease, sleep disturbance and its impacts on emotional and cognitive functioning. She is also active in research on vulnerability and resilience to negative affect in ageing.

**Sascha Callaghan** is a lawyer and lecturer in health law and ethics at the University of Sydney Law School, Australia. She has published widely in the area of healthcare decision-making, mental health and cognitive impairment. She is currently a lead researcher in the Sydney Neuroscience Network and has interests in the intersection between neuroscience, law and ethics.

**Ashley Carr** is a research fellow at the University of Melbourne, Australia, School of Social and Political Sciences, currently researching public perceptions of dementia and the role of regulation in dementia care, under the Cognitive Decline Research Partnership Centre. Research interests include aged and dementia care, social and cultural histories of dementia, and the politics of voice.

**Josephine Clayton** is a Professor of Palliative Care at the University of Sydney, Australia and Director of the HammondCare Centre for Learning and Research in Palliative Care. Her research interests include clinical communication, psycho-oncology, advance care planning and palliative and end-of-life care.

**Sue Field** is an Australian legal practitioner who has researched, taught and practiced in the area of Elder Law for close to 20 years. She is a current member of the New South Wales Law Society's Elder Law, Capacity and Succession Committee, and was a member of the Australian Law Reform Commission's Elder Abuse Advisory Committee. She is an editor for the *Elder Law Review* and a Lead Investigator at the Cognitive Decline Partnership Centre.

**Lynette R. Goldberg** is an academic at the Wicking Dementia Research and Education Centre, Tasmania. She has a background in speech pathology and is a Fellow of the American Speech-Language-Hearing Association. Since 2014, she has focused on dementia education and care through her work as the Coordinator of the Wicking Centre's award-winning Bachelor of Dementia Care programme and her funded research on the difficulties in swallowing, and oral and nutritional health experienced by older adults with dementia. She interacts closely with healthcare staff and understands the critical importance of reframing support and care for people with dementia.

**Irja Haapala** is a senior research fellow at the University of Melbourne, Australia, School of Social and Political Sciences and university lecturer at the

University of Eastern Finland, Department of Educational Science and Teacher Education, currently researching public perceptions of dementia in a three-year project under the Cognitive Decline Research Partnership Centre. Research interests include public health promotion.

**Karen Hutchinson** is a PhD research student with the University of Sydney, Australia, conducting qualitative research into the impact of younger onset dementia (YOD) on self and the family. Research interests include emotional wellbeing of young people and empowerment of young people in families living with YOD.

**Suzanne Jarrad** is a researcher and advocate in the ageing sector and the health arena, with a particular interest in socio-legal issues and quality care. She has recently conducted research into care and job quality in aged care services and the effectiveness of mediation in advance care directive disputes.

**Adele Kelly** is a HammondCare Research Assistant, with a clinical health and research background.

**Susan Kurrle** is a Geriatrician at Hornsby Ku-ring-gai Hospital, New South Wales, Australia and Curran Professor in Health Care of Older People at the University of Sydney, Australia. She is the Director of the Cognitive Decline Partnership Centre and has research interests in dementia care and service development, and elder abuse.

**Gaynor Macdonald** is a social anthropologist, with a focus on how Australian Indigenous peoples have confronted waves of social and cultural change, and the impact of these on their understandings of their personhood and social relationships. In 2013 her husband was diagnosed with Alzheimer's. Taken aback at the lack of insightful and useful support available to carers, she drew on her work on personhood and social stigma to contribute to research into attitudes towards dementia care and carers.

**Tracey McDonald** is Professor and Chair of Ageing at the Australian Catholic University. She is engaged in all aspects of ageing and focuses her research and scholarship on issues affecting older adults; clinician safety and quality; practice-driven research and development; information technology; and life quality. She has experience in social policy, professional clinical practice, education, research and management.

**Jane Mears** is an Associate Professor in the School of Social Sciences and Psychology at Western Sydney University, Australia. She has been researching caring since the mid-1980s, focusing on care and those who devote their lives to caring, care workers, paid and unpaid. She also researches, writes and teaches about ageing, caring, disability and violence prevention. Underpinning her work is a passionate commitment to creating a more caring world.

**Ailin Naderbagi** is a PhD candidate at the University of Sydney, Australia. Her research interests intersect with the themes of this volume with regard to the social, economic and environmental entanglements that problematise ideas of health and wellbeing.

**Andrea D. Price** is a registered nurse, early career academic and lecturer with the Bachelor of Dementia Care (Wicking Dementia Research and Education Centre, University of Tasmania). As a nurse, she worked extensively with older people across a range of clinical settings (including residential aged care, community nursing and mental health), and saw the positive outcomes that are possible from person-centred and relationship-centred approaches to care. Her research is focused on improving the care and support of people with dementia who are living in residential aged care facilities, particularly those who live in dementia-specific units.

**Helen Radoslovich** is employed as the Manager of Growth and Development with Helping Hand Aged Care. She has broad experience in non-government and government roles and as a private consultant. Her current interests are consumer and carer engagement and diversity and inclusion policies within the organisation.

**Pamela Roach** is currently an Adjunct Assistant Professor in the Department of Community Health Sciences at the University of Calgary, Canada, and manages the Brain and Mental Health Research Clinics as part of the Hotchkiss Brain Institute, also at the University of Calgary. She completed her PhD working with families living with young onset dementia, and her postdoctoral research explored family transitions and health expectation in early onset dementia. Her research foci include younger onset dementia, family and patient experiences, qualitative methods and using clinical registry data to improve care provision.

**Chris Roberts** is an Academic General Practitioner in the Faculty of Medicine and Health at the University of Sydney, Australia. His health services research focuses on the impact of complex interventions in primary and community care, including those living with chronic disease. He has a particular interest in inter-professional collaborative practice around aged care for both health-care professional students and graduates. He is currently a co-investigator on a National Health and Medical Research Council project which seeks to enlist general practitioners to engage older people in fall prevention.

**Craig Sinclair** is a research fellow at the Rural Clinical School of Western Australia, with research interests in advance care planning and end-of-life decision-making. He has recently published on a clinical trial of advance care planning, and is currently investigating the views of people with dementia towards supported decision-making.

**Kathy Williams** has lived experience caring for her late mother who had dementia and is involved as a consumer in a number of research activities. She has a Bachelor of Behavioural Studies, majoring in Psychology and Sociology. Working in an ageing policy role, she contributes to government ageing policy and provides high-level strategic, legislative and policy advice to the South Australia Minister for Ageing.

**Gail Yapp** is a HammondCare Research Assistant and works at the University of Technology, Sydney, Australia and is a student at the University of Tasmania (Dementia Care). She has a health and aged care policy background. For this volume, she has worked with colleagues from four universities across Australia who have a common research interest in advance care planning. Collectively they bring extensive experience from a range of areas in the health and aged care sectors: consumer perspective, palliative medicine, psychology, research and policy.

# 1 Reframing dementia

## The social imperative

*Gaynor Macdonald, Jane Mears and
Ailin Naderbagi*

### Dementia as social experience

What we hope to achieve in this book is represented in its title, *Dementia as
Social Experience: Valuing Life and Care.* We challenge the idea that we should
fear dementia or that, once diagnosed, 'life' has virtually come to an end. This
interdisciplinary collection examines how different knowledges and practices
interact, such that they diminish or enhance the lives of those who have been
diagnosed with dementia, as well as those who share their lives. It offers a critique of taken-for-granted ideas and understandings which are found in wider
society, as well as in care practices, while envisioning what it takes to create a
society in which vulnerability is a legitimate, well-supported life experience, and
care is valued as central to all life.

We are not alone in our efforts to reframe dementia. This book draws and
builds on the work of many researchers, activists and policy makers who have
been and are working from a similar perspective. The shifts we are looking for
are not happening fast enough. The medical model and the care industry itself
are major impediments: these are expressions of powerful vested interests. We
seek to reframe dementia: to move an understanding of dementia as a social
experience to centre stage, to be given equal priority to biomedical concerns.
And we seek to dislodge the cultural and medical idea that we are 'individuals',
so as to move towards an appreciation of all human beings as fundamentally
relational beings. More of an impediment to the change that is required,
however, is the lack of a vision for a caring society. To imagine a liveable life
with dementia is, by implication, to imagine a more liveable society, a more
caring society for all citizens. Instead of starting with dementia as a cruel, feared
and vilified disease, let us start with a revaluing of vulnerability and care as
intrinsic to all life.

Dementia is now a well-recognised umbrella term for diseases which produce
cognitive decline. The majority are cases of Alzheimer's disease (70 per cent)
and affect people over the age of 65 years. About 7 per cent are forms of younger
onset dementia. There is readily-available information on the websites of
national dementia organisations about its different forms, typical progressions
and the fact that all forms are, at present, incurable. There are quite regular

announcements of research breakthroughs, as well as lifestyle advice (nutrition and exercise) to help avoid its onset. These chapters do not concern themselves with defining forms of dementia, nor on adding to this wealth of information about the disease and its trajectories. Little of this information assists people *live* with dementia. The brain has no pain receptors and dementia, as a disease of the brain, is quiet and painless: many people go undiagnosed for years. The real impacts – and the need for diagnosis – are felt in relationship. The *experience of dementia is social* – these brain changes affect a person's *behaviour* as the capacity for independent social interaction is impaired.

There is a great need to enhance our capacity to *live with dementia*. We need to give equal value to acquiring the knowledge, skills and attitudes that will improve and enhance this social experience as we give to brain research. Dementia is experienced in interpersonal relationships, by both the person undergoing cognitive decline as well as all those around them: in the small changes that take place over time in a person's capacity to live independently or think clearly, in their need for support, care and empathy or in the requirement on the part of others to understand and to care. As long ago as 1992, Sabat and Harré showed that a social constructionist approach revealed that the self of personal identity persisted into the end stages of Alzheimer's and that the primary cause of its loss is *the ways in which others treat that person*. These social understandings need to come to the fore.

This collection brings together researchers and practitioners who are committed to changing public perceptions, to reframing dementia in ways that challenge the stigma it engenders, so as to provide the conditions for viable enriched lives for all those living with dementia. We use the phrase, 'living with dementia', to refer not only to those who live with a diagnosis of dementia, but to all whose lives are entangled with each diagnosed person: family, friends, colleagues, medical and health professionals, neighbours. Each person living with dementia will experience this entanglement in different ways: each will encounter the stigmas, fears and isolation, and need to deal with the increasing demands for care and consideration that the diagnosed person will require.

Unsettling the dominance of biomedical models, by reframing dementia, does not imply being critical of the enormous energy and commitment going into understanding the neurology of various dementias to find preventive measures, treatments and cures. Rather, it is to say that this is not enough. Until and unless dementia can be prevented and/or cured, we need to learn to live with it. The side-lining of a social model contributes to fear and stigma; these are exacerbated when the medical model is foregrounded. Each diagnosis of dementia impacts on many people. As the disease progresses so, too, do the social demands. We live in societies ill-equipped to deal with these demands, whether for the person with the diagnosis, or those who will care for them as they become progressively dependent, whether at home or in residential care. We need to challenge people who hear a diagnosis of dementia and say, 'how tragic', and encourage them to say, 'how can I support this person and her carers?'.

Reframing *living* with dementia means to move it from a personal medical tragedy to a social issue, one that affects whole families, neighbourhoods and society at large. These chapters, in different ways, affirm the need for a counter narrative to the cognition-centred biomedical framing of dementia. They do not speak with one voice. They take different, sometimes contradictory approaches and, as editors, we believe this is necessary to the debates we must have about how to move forward, whether as a society or in our own interpersonal relationships. We need new ways of thinking and speaking about dementia beyond deficit-based medical framing; a social rather than medical model of dementia, and dementia care must be our starting point if we are to change public perceptions and enhance care giving. More positive models will honour the dignity, experience and wellbeing of the person diagnosed and, by extension, counter narratives will have profound effects for carers and others impacted by the diagnosis.

There are two fronts in this movement for change reflected in these chapters: the need to confront and change social attitudes, which also inform policy and economic decisions; and improvements in the understandings and practices brought to the experience of living with dementia. McDonald (Chapter 2) tackles the first, arguing that it is time for a groundswell of resistance to the negativity surrounding dementia. People in the early stages of dementia, and particularly those diagnosed with early onset dementia, have become more vocal in recent years; they are powerful advocates but they must not be the only voices for change, especially as the change required presents a formidable challenge.

Discussing the need for changes in social attitudes and practices, two recurring themes emerge across these chapters. The first is the negative impact of deep-seated cultural ideas. Authors look critically at the need to reframe social attitudes to address persistent negativity and fear. These social dimensions are complex: they include a history of stigma, fear and misinformation; discrimination linked to ageing; social inequalities; and cultural attitudes about cognition and rationality (McDonald, Mears, Hutchinson *et al.*, Biggs *et al.* and Jarrad, in Chapters 2, 3, 4, 5 and 6, respectively). Understanding the social, historical and ideational contexts of pejorative attitudes assists in challenging them, enabling us to improve the quality of care, which is the second aspect of reframing dementia discussed.

Among these are the notions that, as human beings, we are only of social worth as fully-competent individuals with a certain level of cognitive capacity, which enables us to live what is considered a 'normal' life. Jarrad (Chapter 6) show how reframing dementia can lead to acceptance of different types of 'normality', and to the recognition of experience as an important part of one's quality of life, including the experience of living with dementia. The high bar set for cognitive ability is not, in fact, the reality for many people, at any time in their lives, and some people's greatest strengths are sensual, emotional and relational.

A second theme is the impact of competing economic interests that allocate value according to discriminatory social ideas (especially McDonald and Mears, Chapters 2 and 3, respectively). The reframing required to make life liveable for people with dementia is not only of perceptions and practices specific to the dementia experience; it is needed by us all if we are to live once again in socially-aware and caring societies. The change needed to reframe dementia is going to be tough and it will take time. In the face of what might seem impossible odds, these chapters also examine very practical, often small but meaningful, steps which will work towards achieving this vision of significant social change. Authors examine how to change thinking about practices, attitudes and legislative requirements which impact on the quality of interpersonal relationships (Hutchinson *et al.*, Jarrad, Sinclair *et al.*, Yapp *et al.*, Carr and Biggs and Macdonald, in Chapters 4, 6, 7, 8, 10 and 11, respectively). These discussions seek to better maintain the autonomy and dignity of people with dementia as well as improve approaches to care. The underlying theme is that the changes required to live a good life with dementia are an essential social investment.

## Dementia as burden

In English-speaking nations, people with dementia are often thought of as tragic, having been robbed of life and cast into a slow and traumatising process of losing their personhood. Cancer has been Australia's most feared disease but there are signs dementia is taking over (Fujita *et al.* 2015; SAGA 2016). Efforts have been made by advocacy groups since the 1970s to get Alzheimer's recognised as a medical condition, one that requires proper treatment (Lock 2013: 13). Anthropologist, Margaret Lock (2013: 13) cites neurogeneticist Peter St George-Hyslop's quip, 'Alzheimer's is not that sexy', it is not 'hot like breast cancer or HIV' and, unlike both of these diseases, lobbying efforts fall short when 'affected people cannot speak for themselves'. She notes that, in the United Kingdom, expenditure on dementia is less than 10 per cent of that invested in cancer research. This neglect has been, in large part, because of the stigma associated with the condition. But there are signs of change: 'the concerted efforts of medical professionals, AD societies, and the media to make Alzheimer's more publicly visible as a condition that demands immediate attention for economic, social, and humanitarian reasons are beginning to pay off' (Lock 2013: 13). Money is now being poured into medical research designed to find cures or at least treatments to hold symptoms at bay.

Kevern (2017) maintains that the search for a cure or effective treatment acts as a means of reducing the sense of social fear around the condition, yet arguably it also has the reverse effect, heightening fears because it is a long-term project with uncertain outcomes. While the medical search continues, what needs to be addressed are the fears that can cause those living with dementia to become isolated, relegated to a kind of social death (see Macdonald, Chapter 11). Whether it is the fact that we are living longer, or that lifestyle changes are increasing the incidence, it is how we value the lives of our fellow human beings – from cradle to grave – that must be a primary consideration.

It is not simply the disease, but the way in which people with the disease are treated, that is a fear factor. Dementia is seen as a burden on society. In fact, the societal burden arguably receives more concerned attention than the burden these very attitudes place on those who are at the forefront of the experience of living with dementia. This burden is generally represented as economic, and feeds into ageism. Citizens are divided, into those who 'contribute' (economically) and those who drain the contributions of others, pointing to cultural ideas and values that do not encompass and care for all people. In one Australian survey, 44 per cent of people believed that people with dementia are discriminated against or treated unfairly and, perhaps more disturbingly, 22 per cent indicated that they would feel uncomfortable spending time with someone who had dementia (Phillipson *et al.* 2012: 5). Those who become carers report their own shame and embarrassment about the person they care for: they, too, experience the impact of stigma and public lack of understanding (Phillipson *et al.* 2012: 5). Overcoming stigma, fear, shame, ignorance and denial with regards to dementia are tasks equal in importance and urgency to medical research. We need the knowledge and the tools to equip our societies to live with dementia, to better support those with the dementia diagnosis and those who support them.

In Australia, about 70 per cent of people living with dementia live in their own homes. That is the overwhelming desire for most aged people. But that also means there is no potential for profit as there is in the retirement and residential care sector. The home care workforce is declining, and at the time of writing, early in 2018, there are 100,000 people on the 18-month waiting list for government-funded home care packages (Hermant 2018). At the same time, government funding to residential services, where there are (huge) profits to be made, has increased. Political choices are social choices. By way of example, in 2014, the Australian Federal government (Liberal-National Coalition) implemented 'the most unfair Australian budget in living memory' (Sheil 2014). Spies-Butcher (2014) described it at the time as an attempt to 'fundamentally reshape the social contract. ... It is difficult to see the budget as anything other than an attempt to tear up the social contract and to redistribute income from households and public services to corporations and private business'. It would do so by undermining the reliability and fairness of social security; by undermining institutions designed to promote alternative ideas or enable weaker groups to be heard; and by dismantling public provision to allow greater reliance on private, for-profit businesses.

One justification was the ageing population, yet, as Spies-Butcher (2014) pointed out,

> Australia's pension costs are one of the lowest in the developed world, and will remain one of the cheapest schemes in the future. That's partly because Australia's population is relatively young, and will age relatively slowly. It's also because our pension system is very efficient, targeting those on the lowest incomes.

The 'profound change' actually meant that a social commitment 'to provide equity and security' was being replaced with 'debt and discipline from cradle to grave' (Spies-Butcher 2014). Although public opposition to this budget was intense, that it could be presented at all signals the shift away from social values that is evident in the neoliberal global economy. This makes it imperative that any movement to reinstate social values must start at the grass roots because governments are controlled by high finance rather than social morality. Cutback to social services have been savage, in one country after another. The employment and working conditions of disability and aged care workers are abysmal. Policy looks good but most practice is hideous.

Older people – the 'graying of society' – are now represented as a 'risk' in that they pose an economic challenge (McDonald, Chapter 2). Lock (2013: 13) illustrates how narratives skew attitudes in critiquing reports of dementia. For example, an 'estimated 35.6 million people were living worldwide with dementia in 2010 … estimated to nearly double every 20 years to 65.7 million in 2030 and 115.4 million in 2050'. Such statistics are 'designed to incite political action and increase funding' for dementia research. Concern (negative) is raised about the enormous economic and social burden associated with this phenomenal number of people living with dementia, especially given the small size of most families, because the majority will have to be institutionalised. A concern for the quality of life of those with dementia, and of those who care for them, needs to be at least commensurate with the focus on diagnosis and research into a cure. As Brown (2018) points out, in the United Kingdom (as elsewhere) there is a care crisis, 'a limited social care offering that too often leaves people with dementia footing the bill'. But solving this 'goes beyond throwing money at the situation. Funding is desperately needed, of course, but we can't simply pour more cash into a fundamentally flawed system'. He advocates, as we do, that it is the priorities that need to change. 'Why', he asks, 'does investment in dementia research heavily focus on a cure for future generations, while less than 5% of funding goes to researching the best care possible for all those affected today?' This flawed system needs more attention. It is not just a question of improving 'knowledge and practices among health and social care professionals', although that is important, but of improving 'the quality and inclusivity of the wider system'.

The system needs to transform and incremental modifications or cost cutting approaches will not be enough to address the challenge. Australia needs a model focused on wellness (rather than illness), that has a more integrated, preventive and outcomes-focused approach. New policy, underpinned by real and practical action is needed. In Australia, for example, by 2025, investment of up to an additional $24 billion in capital costs and $13 billion per annum in operating costs would be needed just to meet the projected gaps in residential aged care, community aged care, home and community care and hospital beds. An additional 180,000 carers for the aged care sector will be needed, as well as an extra 85,000 nurses across both the health and ageing sectors. These figures represent just a part of the shortfall in the social infrastructure that supports health and ageing. They take a top-down approach and don't take into account the 'soft' social infrastructure, including the workforce (paid and unpaid), processes, models of care, and payment and funding mechanisms. The shortfall can be read as pointing to a looming budget and political crisis for government, or, to shift the paradigm, as evident of this society's (it is not alone, of course) lack of commitment to the cradle to grave social contract. The politics are demeaning. Statistics are used to identify problems and demands, creating the impression of people who impose this financial 'burden' on others, when it is, rather, an illustration of an uncaring society.

We can change the treatment of those living with dementia and pour more money into their care, but we will not restore liveable lives to them unless, at the same time, we rethink the ways in which dementia is framed within social life. Dementia is not our tragedy. The real tragedy is our historical legacy: the way in which modern western societies have come to conceptualise humanness as individualised substance, to which differential statuses (and, implicitly, differential value) can be attributed. The independent, healthy and wealthy are not 'the norm', there is no 'norm'. Life is full of vicissitudes that we may or may not see coming. If we are social beings, we should be able to live in a society that will uphold us regardless of our circumstances.

## Moving beyond a biomedical view of 'life'

Knowledge about dementia is commonly conveyed in Australia in one of three forms: in the domain of neuroscience as somatic disease; in care industries as a loss of personhood stemming from cognitive decline; and, more recently, as a change in the social demands of relatedness. The key differences in these perspectives are ontological: they stem from differing understandings of what it means 'to be' and what constitutes a 'liveable' life. Thus, they are also moral.

The somatic approach focuses on the human body (soma). In 1906, Dr Alois Alzheimer identified dementia as pertaining to the brain. Prior to his discovery, dementias were understood as problems of the mind. As people became older, it was not unusual that their memory would fade, their 'mind would go' and they would be defined as mad. If too difficult to manage at home, they might be consigned to a lunatic asylum, the only option in the nineteenth century. Alzheimer's significant achievement was to bring people with dementias into the orbit of biomedicine.

The second approach focuses on cognition and what it means to be 'a person'. The idea that cognitive ability is at the heart of 'being human' means that dementia, defined as cognitive decline, is stigmatised as loss – loss of self, of personhood, of mind, of independence. A third approach is relational. Dementia makes distinctive claims on relationship, as do many other challenging life experiences (parenting, a new work environment, a disability). Each of these perspectives contains important insights but it is where the emphasis is placed that has implications for understanding how to live with dementia and how we should develop care practices.

Efforts to wrest public images away from madness to understanding dementia as disease are ongoing; dementias still carry the weight of the stigma and prejudice associated with 'mental' illnesses, those that do not have a clear biomedical (somatic) basis. Yet, in part, this is a problem of the medical model itself; its dominance does not allow space for socially-oriented understandings. The medical model of dementia understands it as 'a matter of biochemical processes and mechanisms internal to brains gone awry' (Moser 2011: 710). A somatic understanding 'shapes life with dementia as a more or less given disease trajectory in which the subjective and agential "I" of the patient is progressively broken down and eradicated', leading to 'a process of progressive separation, isolation, individualization, and disconnection from practices and interactions, whether at home or within residential care' (Moser 2011: 715). But this is only a mode of ordering knowledge and experience about dementia.

There has recently been a significant shift within the somatic approach. While the implications of the interaction of our genes and our environment are readily granted with regard to disease causation, environmental variables in the cases of dementia have been seen as beyond the ken of biomedical researchers and research efforts remain predominantly focused on molecular changes. Social and political factors are increasingly coming to the fore in a paradigm shift that has seen the focus on finding a cure move towards discovering preventative measures. Research on prevention continues the reductionist focus on internal molecular changes in the body. A major reason being, as Lock (2013: 8) points out, that this serves the interests of the pharmaceutical industry. The shift is designed to assess who is at risk from dementia, with the aim of developing means to intercede at the 'prodromal stage', perhaps 20 years before clinical symptoms in the form of behavioural changes can be detected (Lock 2012: 297).

Different modes of understanding enable us to act upon and enact dementia in different ways and only a social mode can help shape more positive ways of *living* with dementia. This is something the medical model provides no clues about. Kate Swaffer (2017), diagnosed at the age of 49 years, and now an inspiring advocate, illustrates what happens when people with dementia are cast into this dark, medicalised space when she observes that,

> the health sector is currently still providing 'late stage' management of dementia for people more often now being diagnosed in the earlier stages. I may have been diagnosed with dementia, but frankly there was no point taking on an assumed death that day.

Hutchinson and colleagues (Chapter 4) argue that the medical model focuses on deficits, on what people living with dementia cannot do or are not. We need to embrace a can-do approach, a social model focused on everyday life. It is difficult to reframe services and support to be socially-responsive and aware when they are defined and dominated by a medical model whose starting point is negative. This is not just an issue for those with younger onset dementia; people do not have to be 'written off' because they are diagnosed in later life either.

Debilitating attitudes remain evident among medical and health professionals. This is particularly concerning as these are the people who should be leading the changes and demanding social and economic investment. While among the general population there is an evident lack of awareness of what dementia is and its impacts (Biggs *et al.*, Chapter 5), there is little excuse for misinformation and patronising attitudes within health arenas. As Jarrad (Chapter 6) illustrates, professionals continue to de-enable because of their own prejudices and stereo-types. This points to poor training.

The significant benefits that emerge from a re-orientation in the training of professionals is evident in the chapter by Goldberg and colleagues (Chapter 9). They explicitly develop a biopsychosocial model in training, focused on the person not the diagnosis. Importantly, it encourages self-reflection on the part of students, enhancing their appreciation of the changes in their own attitudes and behaviours that are necessary to good dementia care. Intended for those who provide direct care to people with dementia, this chapter emphasises the need for adopting a 'personhood lens' to enable caregivers to understand and provide the quality of care that supports and assists people with dementia to remain socially engaged. They point out the need for a transition in care work from a reactive behaviour management approach, to a proactive approach which aims at preserv-ing the dignity of the person. This would have far reaching benefits in reducing the stigma and power imbalances faced by people living with dementia, as well as optimising their quality of life. Importantly, they demonstrate the ways in which caregivers' attitudes are transformed through good education. Their learn-ings from student caregivers should become widely disseminated across the entire sector, incorporated into the training of all doctors, nurses, allied-health professionals and professional caregivers, from medical degrees to certificates in aged care.

## Social and cultural factors standing in the way of change

As a part of the awareness required to bring about attitudinal change, McDonald (Chapter 2) highlights the capacity of words for creating a dominant narrative about a particular issue, thus shaping the social and political attitudes and judge-ments around it. The conventional narratives that develop can not only act as a barrier for new and diverse understandings about the issue in question, but also be used in strategic ways for certain gains. Dementia is one space where the power of dominant narratives is clearly evident. McDonald refers to this 'neg-ative positioning' as a form of abuse, rooted in ageism. She highlights how an older person's natural responses of feeling distressed, frustrated or depressed about a situation over which they feel they have no control can be exploited by those around them, through strategically retelling the narrative for personal gain and in the worst cases dispossessing someone from their assets. Jarrad's (Chapter 6) chapter gives a distressingly poignant example.

Raising social awareness and changing dominant narratives about ageing and dementia with more empowering frameworks will be crucial in moving towards reducing ageist abuse and building capacity for equitable resource distribution. Jarrad also states the need for a counter narrative to the cognition-centred bio-medical framing of dementia which foregrounds deficit, to one that honours the dignity, experience and wellbeing of the person diagnosed. By extension, counter narratives will have profound effects for carers (see Hutchinson *et al.*, Chapter 4).

In the background, and often the foreground of negative attitude, is ageism. Ageism is one reason why social investment in changing attitudes to ageing – and thus to dementia – is low. In interrogating this issue, both McDonald (Chapter 2) and Mears (Chapter 3) examine how, as a form of discrimination, ageism creates inequities by affecting access to public health resources, financial security and legal protection for people impacted by dementia as patients or carers. McDonald refers to the negative positioning of dementia, rooted in ageism, as a form of abuse. The stereotypical narratives around dementia in broader society enable this repositioning of the behaviour of the elderly person in negative terms in order to convince others to accept their version as legitimate. Mears' focus on older women shows how they bear the burden of ageist and sexist discrimination and inequity in particularly harsh ways.

McDonald (Chapter 2) argues that elder abuse is the third part of a triptych of abuses, alongside domestic violence and child abuse, that are occurring within trust relationships. Governments, businesses and social leaders, including the media, are well positioned to lead the type of social change that has begun to curtail domestic violence and paedophilia in recent times. They must focus the insights learnt on changing negative attitudes to the aged: reframing dementia will play a major part in this. In an economic system that values self-interest and competition, negative positioning arises in a large part from prejudice or competition for resources. It is well-recognised that acceptance of people living with disability requires positive repositioning of attitudes and values: events such as the Paralympics help achieve this. The same effort must go into changing attitudes for those living with mental illness, mental confusion and dementias. Strategies for raising awareness of ageism and its consequences have been developed in Australia, along with several reports on human rights and systematic abuse of older people's rights but, as Mears (Chapter 3) shows, translating this wisdom into outcomes for older people, particularly those with dementia, is yet to occur. Ageism within families and societies is a clear target area for prevention of all types of abuse and improving personal security.

The feminisation of ageing and the intersecting of age and gender have significant implications for dementia research and the development of policy and practice. We need to identify the social structures and processes that lead to a silencing of the gendered implications of dementia, thus exacerbating disadvantage. Discussions about dementia pay scant attention to the wealth of lived experiences held by women, who form a diverse yet under-researched and often silenced group. A focus on gender in the context of dementia will better enable researchers and activists to understand the power relationships that promote ageism and abuse, to engage meaningfully with older women not just to ensure their voices are heard, but so that they are involved in devising and influencing research programmes, policies and practices. Mears (Chapter 3) argues that, through an understanding of power and gender, and using a framework that challenges the intersectionality of ageism and sexism, we can think through ways to bring about social justice and social change.

Attitudes towards older people and dementia are not, however, uniformly held. Increased media attention and public debate raises the issue of how dementia is perceived. Social responses to dementia are becoming increasingly important, including the effects of fear of dementia. Biggs and colleagues (Chapter 5) use the framework of generational intelligence to demonstrate how people with dementia are 'othered' differently according to age, with some surprising differences across age brackets. Their approach shows how a renewed focus on positive othering, which can recognise differences as well as commonalities between age groups and phenomena associated with age, may help the better recognition and valorising of ageing, disease and associated experiences. This would form a first step to better public education so as to bridge divides between generations and enhance the positive adoption of public health messages, and ultimately, social adaptation to dementia.

Much of the negativity about dementia stems from cultural values. Jarrad (Chapter 6), concerned with autonomy and decision-making on the part of vulnerable older people, offers a critique of the liberal idea of autonomy as the governing of self by a reasoning individual, arguing that autonomous decision-making in the case of advanced dementia is necessarily relational. The quality of daily life, and a vulnerable person's sense of autonomy and capacity, is enhanced or diminished by the attitudes and behaviours of those with whom that person is in relationship.

The pervasive ideal of the person as a rational individual has led, under neoliberalism, to what Post (2000) calls a 'hypercognitive' society. Those who do not meet this threshold, as in the case of dementia, become lesser persons, socially and legally. The attitudes that stem from this are powerful in damaging a person's sense of self, their confidence and ability to exercise autonomy, further constraining their options and choices. As Jarrad (Chapter 6) argues, this cognitive approach also ignores the essential contribution of values, emotions and intuition in enabling individuals to determine personal priorities in decision-making (see Sinclair *et al.* and Yapp *et al.*, Chapters 7 and 8, respectively). In this sense, the determination of capacity should be a last resort instead of a starting point. The legal construct of capacity can disadvantage someone in a medical setting, where relational, person-centred approaches are better able to respect autonomy. We need to move from the traditional view of dementia as a 'loss of self' to an understanding that the person with dementia is experiencing their disability as the 'new normal', and open up possibilities of enhancing functioning through 'strength-based approaches' (Jarrad, Chapter 6). This requires a broader understanding of 'the person' as multi-dimensional, not defined solely by cognitive ability. In exploring alternative approaches to decision-making beyond the capacity approach, a person-centred model that respects the whole person and their life meaning is required (Macdonald, Chapter 11).

Successful initiatives that are changing discriminations, vulnerabilities and abuse include the advance care directives discussed by Sinclair *et al.* (Chapter 7) and Yapp *et al.* (Chapter 8). They focus on the need to shift the emphasis in advance care planning from an end-of-life medical model, to a rest-of-life model. Initially developed within the hospital context to address medical treatment decisions and the documentation in advance of consent or refusal of treatments, advance care planning should be reframed as a process of discussion about goals and values relating to future care for and by the people living with dementia. These authors show the benefits of a positive positioning of advance care planning, focused on living as opposed to dying, shaped by personal, familial and cultural values.

The notion of the autonomous self who makes their own rational decisions, independent of the relational contexts in which they live, forms the neoliberal image of the ideal citizen (Carr and Biggs, Jarrad and Macdonald, Chapters 10, 8 and 11, respectively). This is challenged when autonomous decision-making is positioned in *relational* terms. Authors in this volume reveal another common thread: increasingly, researchers and practitioners are seeing that decision-making is not an individual act, nor one operating on the basis of rational cost-benefit analysis. Rather, it is grounded in an environment of social relatedness, with all the challenges and benefits that this presents.

Taking up the conceptual framework of dyadic coping theory and relational autonomy, Sinclair and colleagues (Chapter 7) examine the ways stressors in the context of dementia may be interdependently appraised and acknowledged as shared, because this impacts the experience of decision-making. Decision-making as a stressor is significantly affected by fear of social impacts. Coping configurations are constantly in flux, shifting as the dementia progresses and the relationships involved have to change. A framing of decision-making as relational enables more sensitivity to the range of factors that influence how situations are appraised and decisions made by all concerned. Concern for values associated with maintaining the integrity of relationships implicated in decision-making, and taking account of issues faced by carers, must be central in designing interventions and support programmes that better suit the experiences of those involved and enable adaptive responses.

Autonomy is a major theme because it points to the integrity of each person, and requires that we focus on the abilities, rights and dignity of others. Misdiagnosis (deliberate and unintended), self-interest, lack of forward planning and lack of consideration are all reasons that autonomy is ignored, and thus are reasons for its importance. Jarrad (Chapter 6) does point out, however, that respect for autonomy is a challenge in the face of progressive cognitive impairment. In the broadest sense, to act in a self-determining way is understood to be the expression of a person's internal thoughts, values and emotions, which comprise their unique sense of self in response to their exterior world. This requires that person's voice to be heard, their needs and desires to be interpreted even when they may have difficulty communicating. In part this can be accomplished with some knowledge of a person's history and the context in which they are at the time, linking back to what Carr and Biggs (Chapter 10) stress about relationship: relationships shape a person's sense of self and their capacity to adapt.

This can be enabled or disabled by carers. To provide for a person's autonomy means to create the environment, practices and relationships that maximise a sense of self and wellbeing.

Hutchinson *et al.* (Chapter 4) examine the theme of invisibility which creates experiences of isolation, discrimination and marginalisation for all members of a family living with dementia, in particular where there are children and young people directly affected when a member is diagnosed with younger onset dementia. It can be difficult to maintain meaningful relationships and connections when lives deviate from their expected trajectory because of a dementia diagnosis. Although focused on younger families, these insights have broad application. They demonstrate the ways in which inadequate approaches from service providers can be socially and psychically disabling.

As Carr and Biggs (Chapter 10) point out, autonomy is also important to the quality of a work environment for care workers and can be denied by an over-zealous focus on regulation which can inhibit the kinds of approaches they may wish to take. They show the dilemmas for care workers who have to juggle regulations and workplace demands that effectively prevent meaningful connection. Sometimes this works in their favour, as they can use regulations to protect themselves from overload, but thus works against those who should be in receipt of their attention. The demands these authors identify are exacerbated, of course, by inadequate staffing levels, which are common across the aged care industry.

To see people as relational beings is not to subsume them into an amorphous 'social'. On the contrary, it enhances the presence and contribution of each person within any given situation. On a ward, for example, this might include patients, visitors, nursing staff, cleaners, social workers, physiotherapists, doctors – all of whom might be present in a situation at the same time. But it does make one aware that each of these people is impacting, in some way, on every other person, whether knowingly or not. There will be power and knowledge differentials, perhaps creating hierarchies, gender and age dynamics, personality issues and so on. Some people will feel affirmed, others invisible or demeaned. What connections are being made, or not, are affecting the wellbeing of each person in that situation.

Macdonald (Chapter 11) argues for a major paradigm shift and focuses attention on the 'real experts', the people with knowledge, understanding and experience of caring for (and about) those with dementia. In also critiquing neoliberal and biomedical framings of dementia, she underlines the substantial gaps this leaves in dealing with the social aspects of dementia, which inevitably connect to quality of relationship. She also calls for a relational approach to dementia and care, as well as the need to recognise and privilege the 'common sense' knowledge of those at the coalface: family carers who constantly face the challenge to change and adapt to the vicissitudes of dementia despite the lack of positive resources and support in the broader community wherein care remains an undervalued undertaking. The paradigm shift can be achieved, it is in everybody's interest and should be everybody's business.

These chapters do not suggest that changing attitudes and practices will be easy. However, they send two messages. One is the enormous work that has already been put into imagining and working towards change; and the other is an acknowledgement of the enormity of the task ahead. These chapters are grounded in qualitative research and real-life experience; hence they are also practical, examining the kinds of practices that can be rethought or reoriented in order to make change happen. The focus is on interpersonal change, which is fundamental to changes at the level of institutions, government policy and programmes.

There are now successful community-based programmes, such as the Welsh town of Brecon's dementia-friendly initiative. Edinburgh, Scotland has declared itself a dementia-friendly city: various local level initiatives are encouraged and supported throughout the city, with the initiative promoted on the City of Edinburgh Council's website. Their 'dementia stigma leaflet' aptly begins by stating, 'We can't cure dementia yet but we can all cure the stigma'. With the right attitudes, change is possible. However, Edinburgh is an exception. Most of these initiatives, as in the case of Brecon, have been started and run by community activists, not professionals or government actors. This is also the case in Australia, where the town of Kiama has taken a lead but others have been slow to follow. This highlights the need for changes in societal attitudes, a task which cannot be left solely to local people.

## Dementia care as relational care

Perhaps what is really frightening about dementia is that we fear both the loss of control over our lives and also the knowledge that we may not be cared for as we would wish. Despite the fact that the number of people living with dementia is increasing, and the majority of them are living within the community, in their own homes, there is a significant imbalance between the research that focuses on experiences of people living with dementia and their carers in the community, as compared with the much greater focus on the experiences of those in residential care homes. In part, this is a question of access: those in residential care are easier to target, and the care industry has resources not available to those living in their own homes. Unfortunately, as mentioned above, it has a lot to do with cost and whether or not there is a profit to be made.

Research is only just beginning to be conducted on how relationality impacts on the quality of care. One example is a study being conducted to examine the relationship and wellbeing of both the older parent and their children:

> Most aged care studies track either the carer or the care recipient, but not both. And yet, it's the interaction between the adult child and older parent that is critical in understanding how care is provided, how it's received, and how parents and children influence one another's wellbeing.
> (Gery Karantzas, cited in Community Care Review Staff Writers, 2018)

In the context of dementia, it is taken for granted that care will become too much of a burden for those at home and that residential care is inevitable. The diagnosis of dementia is replete with messages of loss, and this loss of control is but one. At the same time, Australians continue to see nursing homes as places of antiseptic neglect, depersonalisation and loss of dignity, to be avoided at all costs. Improving care in these homes would certainly attract clients. A recent study (Murphy and Ibrahim 2018) found that the rates of depression and suicide, particularly among male residents, by far exceeds the average for those of similar age not in such homes. Among their recommendations, which include change at a national policy level to lift the overall quality of aged care, is a call for family and friends to play their part in maintaining their loved ones' social connections and feelings of being valued. Sadness, loneliness, feelings of isolation and becoming withdrawn are not, they stress, signs of ageing.

Carr and Biggs (Chapter 10) seek to reframe the care relationship by drawing together the person-centred care and emotional labour literatures to develop a puzzle approach to care. The care worker must combine empathic understanding and professional distancing to solve the puzzles that dementia and dementia care present, in meaningful and rewarding ways. This reframes 'dementia-related behaviours' and care interactions along social and cultural lines: care becomes a set of intelligible responses to a range of factors that demand solutions. These authors' insights could be built upon to enable primary carers at home to think about how they cope as well. Presenting the changing behaviours of people with dementia as a puzzle, to be unravelled and pieced together, lends itself to a problem-solving approach that recognises the importance of the carer's initiative and responses.

The very term 'challenging behaviours', so frequently used in medical models to describe the 'symptoms' of dementia, is an example of how language and modelling can reverse the actual situation. Symptoms once thought to result from neuropathological damage, are now better understood as hard to read reactions to what can be complex situations (see Jarrad, Chapter 6 and Macdonald's comments on agitation, for example in Chapter 11). The 'challenge' for a person with dementia is to get the other person to understand what they want or need. The chapter by Hutchinson and colleagues (Chapter 4) forcibly argues that it is not cognitive impairment that leads to feelings of intra-family and social invisibility but *the reactions of others*. Their behaviour is a challenge *for others*. The onus is on that other, whether a carer or in some other capacity, to solve the puzzle. This is why dementia is always a social experience and cannot be individualised as a medical one. What every person with dementia needs is care givers prepared to take the time to solve the puzzle that being in relationship requires. Thus, dementia as 'catastrophe' can be reframed as 'biographical disruption', requiring adjustment, accommodation and reconciliation on the part of others. The demands this makes on relationships can be intense, but they are made all the more so by the lack of research into how carers might be enabled to recognise and solve these puzzles.

Hutchinson and colleagues (Chapter 4) also point to the need for greater self-awareness on the part of professional carers and support workers to help them adopt a more enabling approach, improving interactions with families and providing greater job satisfaction. But it is easy to criticise the quality of care in a social arena in which it is poorly resourced and remunerated. It is important, as Mears (Chapter 3), Macdonald (Chapter 11) and Goldberg *et al.* (Chapter 9) note, to recognise that caregivers also need to be treated with consideration, respect and dignity. Like these authors, Carr and Biggs (Chapter 10) reveal added dimensions to the relational quality of the care engagement: neither patient nor care worker are privileged. Both are important to the quality of experience and outcome for each person in the relationship.

Contributors examine the importance of person-centred approaches to care but move the reader beyond some of the triteness of this phrase to the growing awareness that person-centred care must preserve autonomy within *relationship*, offering practical approaches that primary carers at home and other family members should be aware of, as well as advice for professional care staff. Evident in these chapters are the demands made on family members, not only those who become carers but also, for example, young people and children in the family. Hutchinson *et al.* (Chapter 4) use a social model of disability to demonstrate that the disabling experiences of people with younger-onset dementia and their carers and family members, is created by the social environment of medical professionals, service providers and the broader community. A social model provides a generative framework that transforms stigma through experientially-informed discussion and education. It enables people to recreate their lives by shifting how the diagnosis is conceptualised, implicitly resisting the negative discourses, as well as demanding more appropriate service provision. There is a significant need for people with dementia and their families to be involved in redesigning service delivery, an involvement which inevitably affects the development of generational intelligence among a myriad of other positive benefits (Biggs *et al.*, Chapter 5).

The differences between patient-centred, person-centred and relational care are significant even while they might appear similar. In this sense, the contributions in this book are imaginative and visionary, pointing forward positively both in their examination of tested, grounded thinking about care approaches and practices, and in conceptual and political challenges. Central to all of them is a critical conversation around personhood and social value. The idea of person-centred care has been around for some decades and has become a largely taken for granted approach. But, as Carr and Biggs (Chapter 10), and Macdonald (Chapter 11) discuss, there has been little critique of the concept and its application. These chapters, as well as those of Goldberg and colleagues (Chapter 9) and Jarrad (Chapter 6), push the boundaries of person-centred care to examine it *in relationship*. What unites understandings of person-centred care is that attention must be given to the person 'hidden' behind cognitive decline (Carr and Biggs, Chapter 10). Goldberg and colleagues look to a transition in care work from a reactive behaviour management approach, to a proactive approach which aims at preserving the dignity of the person. This would have far reaching benefits in reducing the stigma and power imbalances faced by people living with dementia, as well as optimising their quality of life.

One extension of the notion of person-centred care is that of personalisation. Sanderson and Bailey (2013) define personalisation as observing, listening to and understanding what gives a person hope, enjoyment and meaning in their everyday life, in order to tailor care and support to help them either attain or retain these. As Macdonald (Chapter 11) points out, such extensions do not include the carer in a relationship, only in a (personalised) task-oriented way. Admonishing carers to see the person and not the dementia misses the point. The carer is always, as is any person present in a given situation at a given time, in a relationship, and that relationship is constituting the person of the carer at the same time as it is constituting the person of the patient. Think, for example, of the doctor's visit to the ward, perhaps surrounded by students and nurses. His or her demeanour, tone and capacity for a good connection will influence the feelings, behaviours and responses of the person-as-patient, just as the hierarchies of power, knowledge and attitude are constituting the relations among the staff in that situation.

## Reframing dementia

The medicalisation of dementia and the frenzied search for the cure, however desirable and necessary, risks avoiding the conversation we need to have: what is 'life' about and how should we live it well? How we think of ourselves and others, how social value is determined and how this changes over the life course are shaped by ideas embedded in cultural values that are deep-seated and usually taken-for-granted. This is not the place to review either the western history of ideas or other traditions. Suffice it to say that people also think of themselves as *social selves* – particularly outside the modern industrial west – as bound to and influenced by each other in relations of mutual interdependency. A relational approach to understanding dementia and care builds on this notion that all humans, irrespective of cultural beliefs, are inherently constituted through relatedness. It has been shown that we can change attitudes towards gender, disability, the ethnic other – albeit the struggle is ongoing. We can bring similar insights to thinking about the life cycle, including ageing; the experiences of vulnerability that beset everyone; our inherent interdependencies; and our mortality. Dementia brings all these life challenges to the fore; inviting us to rethink ourselves as interdependent, relational beings.

People with dementia are citizens in society, regardless of the setting in which they receive support and care. To say that each person is unique, and that they should be treated with dignity, respect and appropriate autonomy, applies as much to the people in our social circles and workplaces as it does to a person in a residential aged care facility. But in the latter case, it is even more essential with regards to a person who, by definition of their diagnosis, is potentially more vulnerable. They require care and attention that is compassionate and culturally safe. Their social engagement should decrease their vulnerability to stigma and discrimination. Dementia education and training programs need to reflect this approach to care. The chapter by Goldberg *et al.* (Chapter 9) demonstrates that change is possible, person by person. Comments by students who learnt to reframe dementia and its care suggest that terms such as 'person-centred care' are hardly relevant when this is an orientation to life and others. The term points to what has been lost in modern societies, but the opportunity to regain a relational perspective is clearly achievable.

It is unfortunate that we are creating an idea that there is a 'care industry' in which there are 'consumers'. We need to avoid the way in which the notion of 'care' is producing a dual society, wherein those with dependencies are treated one way, and those who are apparently defined as non-dependent are represented as the privileged normal. This duality is also fundamentally gendered. The economist, the manager and the academic are also dependent, vulnerable, human beings. Cartesian ontology and individualism not only deny the legitimacy of our dependencies and vulnerabilities, they privilege the male-focused norms and devalue 'care' activities, representing them as non-productive, female, soft options. Productivity is not the essence of humanness. We are humanly and socially-devalued to the extent that we deny the normalcy of dependency: there are frequent constraints, short- and long-term, on the ways life is lived. Few of them in fact disconnect us. Dementia does not require, and is not, disconnection. But, as Macdonald (Chapter 11) argues, it does demand new ways of understanding what it means to be in connection.

A decade ago, Michael Fine (2007) identified the various contours of the debates about care that had been going on throughout the twentieth century. He highlighted the influence of feminists, such as Carol Gilligan, which had led to work on the ethics of care. Women were the carers and bore the burden of a society's lack of commitment and concern for carers (see a current overview in Barnes and Brannelly 2015). We can see that, if anything, things have become worse for women, especially older women (Mears, Chapter 3). The caring society remains elusive. We want to affirm and acknowledge those who are the true experts in this field, those who are caring or have cared for those with dementia. And we want to thank those with the dementia diagnosis for increasingly being prepared to speak out and demand the changes we need. In different ways, these are the people who are working to create a society that does truly care and value us all.

## References

Barnes, M., T. Brannelly, 2015, *Ethics of Care: Critical Advances in International Perspectives*, Bristol, UK: Policy Press.

Brown, D., 2018, Dementia research must study care as well as cure. *Guardian* (Aust), 19 February 2018, www.theguardian.com/social-care-network/2018/feb/19/dementia-research-cure-care [Accessed 06 March 2018].

Community Care Review Staff Writers., 2018, Link between family relationships and care outcomes under the spotlight, *Community Care Review*, 01 February 2018, www.australianageingagenda.com.au/2018/02/01/link-family-relationships-care-outcomes-spotlight/ [Accessed 04 March 2018].

Fine, M.D., 2007, *A Caring Society?: Care and the Dilemmas of Human Service in the Twenty-First Century*, New York: Palgrave Macmillan.

Fujita, K., H. Sasaki, Y. Kaneko, A. Eboshida, Y. Motohashi, 2015, The impact of cognitive decline and fear of dementia on mental health of elderly people, *The Gerontologist*, 55: 707–708.

Hermant, N., 2018, Government scrambles to respond to growing queue for home-care packages, *ABC News*, 03 February 2018, www.abc.net.au/news/2018-02-03/govt-scrambles-amid-growing-queue-for-home-care-packages/9387692 [Accessed 05 March 2018].

Kevern, P., 2017, Why are we so afraid of dementia, *The Conversation*, 12 September 2017, https://theconversation.com/why-are-we-so-afraid-of-dementia-83175 [Accessed 12 January 2018].

Lock, M., 2012, The epigenome and nature/nurture reunification: A challenge for anthropology, *Medical Anthropology*, 32: 291–308.

Lock, M., 2013, *The Alzheimer Conundrum: Entanglements of Dementia and Aging*, Princeton, USA: Princeton University Press.

Moser, I., 2011, Dementia and the limits to life: Anthropological sensibilities, STS interferences, and possibilities for action in care, *Science, Technology and Human Values*, 36(5): 704–722.

Murphy, B., J. Ibrahim, 2018, Too many Australians living in nursing homes take their own lives, *The Conversation*, 06 March 2018, https://theconversation.com/too-many-australians-living-in-nursing-homes-take-their-own-lives-92112 [Accessed 06 March 2018].

Phillipson, L., C. Magee, S. Jones, E. Skladzien, 2012, Exploring dementia and stigma beliefs: A pilot study of Australian adults aged 40 to 65 years, paper 28, *Alzheimer's Australia*. www.dementia.org.au/files/20120712_US_28_Stigma_Report.pdf [Accessed 06 May 2018].

Post, S., 2000, The concept of Alzheimer Disease in a hypercognitive society, in P.J. Whitehouse, K. Maurer and J.F. Ballenger (eds), *Concepts of Alzheimer Disease: Biological, Clinical, and Cultural Perspectives*, pp. 245–256, Baltimore, USA: Johns Hopkins University Press.

Sabat, S.R., R. Harré, 1992, The construction and deconstruction of self in Alzheimer's disease, *Ageing and Society*, 12: 443–461.

SAGA, 2016, Dementia more feared than cancer new Saga Survey reveals, *SAGA Press Releases*, May 2016, www.saga.co.uk/newsroom/press-releases/2016/may/older-people-fear-dementia-more-than-cancer-new-saga-survey-reveals.aspx [Accessed 08 May 2018].

Sanderson, H., G. Bailey, 2013, *Personalisation and Dementia: A Guide for Person-Centred Practice*, London: Jessica Kingsley.

Sheil, C., 2014, Abbott, Piketty and the spirit of the times, *Journal of Australian Political Economy*, 17 June 2014, http://australianpe.wixsite.com/japehome/single-post/2014/6/17/Abbott-Piketty-and-the-Spirit-of-the-Times [Accessed 03 March 2018].

Spies-Butcher, B., 2014, Debt and discipline from cradle to grave, *Journal of Australian Political Economy*, 25 May 2014, http://australianpe.wixsite.com/japehome/single-post/2014/5/25/Debt-and-Discipline-from-Cradle-to-Grave [Accessed 03 March 2018].

Swaffer, K., quoted in, Staff writer, News Corp Australia, 2017, Diagnosed with dementia Kate Swaffer actively supports people suffering from the same ailment, *Daily Telegraph*, 25 January 2017, www.dailytelegraph.com.au/lifestyle/aotd/diagnosed-with-dementia-kate-swaffer-actively-supports-people-suffering-from-the-same-ailment/news-story/88b326cc7c64fe9325a05875f11960a1 [Accessed 06 May 2018].

# Part I

# Challenging social constructions of ageing and dementia

# 2    Negative positioning of 'dementia' in an environment of competition for resources

*Tracey McDonald*

## Introduction

In social environments driven by self-interest and individualism, people experiencing dementia must compete with others for access to public health resources, legal protection and financial security. Competition for access to resources is a feature of everyday life in most contemporary neoliberal economies (Burt 1993). The idea that competitive self-interest is natural to human beings has informed and justified economic policy; it was described by Schwartz (1986) as 'the cardinal human motive'. This notion of 'economic man' is subject to significant critique, particularly in economic anthropology, but its ideological status persists. In societies increasingly motivated by individualism and material self-interest, the acquisition processes related to material wealth and power have been styled as rational choices rather than as outright competition with others (Miller 1999). Behaviours in pursuit of self-interest in many societies are regarded as being appropriate, sensible and progressive, with the choices of those adopting such strategies continually reinforced as they compete to acquire material and other benefits.

This idea of self-interest impacts in specific ways on the circumstances facing those living with dementia-causing conditions. Within most societies today, adults would be aware of the growing numbers of people affected by cognitive decline or mental confusion, frequently referred to as 'dementias'. In this chapter, I argue that ageism plays a crucial role in the allocation of resources and determines how competing interests may use other people's disadvantage to their own benefit. It epitomises abuses of power and inequality, discrimination, marginalisation and structural violence that promotes vulnerability to attack and endorses an uneven playing field.

Robert Butler (2005) coined the term 'ageism' in 1969 to describe discrimination based on age. It occurs when negative attitudes and demeaning practices are shown towards older people (Angus and Reeve 2006: 138). The influential nature of ageism cannot be dismissed as a factor in the hurdles faced by older people. In any society, old age can be considered a success or failure depending on the extent to which ageism has influenced the culture (McDonald 2012). Indicators of a society's ageist tendencies lie in whether the elderly population is regarded as a normal part of the social make-up or an unintended consequence of policies that have led to population ageing, as reflected in changed national populations where longevity and low birth rates alter the demographic profile. Strategies adopted by those striving towards accumulating wealth and control include negative positioning, misinformation and coercion, all enabled by normalised ageist values within the family, community and society. Nowhere are these dynamics more evident than in the context of dementia.

Public awareness of the concept 'dementia' does not translate into consistency of understanding about possible causes of dementia symptoms, its treatment and even whether the condition is avoidable or reversible with appropriate action. Widespread ignorance about dementia has undermined the quality of discussion and rendered the concept vulnerable to conjecture and misinformation, often spread by those with self-serving agendas. Consequently, the various ways in which 'dementia' has been conceptualised encourages those predisposed to prejudicial thinking to select the model most convenient to their purposes from the array. Some of these are provided in the table below.

There are many other conceptualisations of dementia, but the central idea across these categories is that the word 'dementia' is a powerful explanatory narrative. Some words, because of a general perception of what the word means, convey an idea that prompts immediate 'understanding' of its scope and consequences. The power of the word is generated by the cultural concerns attached to the narrative that springs immediately to mind on hearing it (Mcadams 2006). The words used to direct attention to a topic are able to tap into a general understanding about it, bringing it into awareness. When we rely on a single word to achieve this effect, and assume that the meaning is well understood, the risk of

*Table 2.1* Some social conceptualisations of dementia

| Dementia categorised as: | Dementia seen as: |
| --- | --- |
| Tragedy | • a heartbreaking catastrophe<br>• an identity-absorbing sub-culture<br>• stigmatising |
| Comedy | • a source of mirth and entertainment |
| Opportunity | • lucrative business option<br>• an early access to inheritance<br>• a mechanism to bring out the best in people |
| Risky | • inevitable consequence of long life<br>• inherited from parents<br>• able to be 'caught' from others<br>• a convenient or lazy diagnosis<br>• vulnerability to exploitation and abuse |
| Malice | • label used to denigrate and dominate others<br>• justification for dismissing human rights<br>• reducing competitive advantage |

entrenching inaccuracies and setting up barriers to new information is enhanced. Along with the perception of dementia that is triggered can come a judgement about the person living with the condition. Such judgements have an immediate effect on others: the ongoing value of the person, perhaps also the burdens that someone who is confused may impose on others. For example, the term 'challenging behaviours' is used to categorise the actions of confused and agitated people because they challenge those close by.

The spectrum of interpretations of 'dementia' shown in Table 2.1 suggests that the narrative can be manipulated in strategic ways within cultures and subgroups to produce a pre-determined effect. Strategic narratives are geared to establishing intellectual supremacy over complex ideas that can subsequently be used to gain political or competitive advantage. Once established, strategic narratives can influence general perceptions of an idea in terms of investment worthiness and social acceptance, as well as many other social, economic and political outcomes. Miskimmon and O'Loughlin (2014) refer to this activity as wielding 'soft power' and suggest that public portrayals of ideas can be better understood within such a frame.

## Understanding dementia

In order to better understand a concept as complex as 'dementia' we need to acknowledge that it is currently framed in ways that have different meanings depending on a specific conceptualisation. A person's perceptions of another's dementia symptoms are constructed from a personal information base, values and priorities, and even private agendas. In some instances, these symptoms can appear humorous: skilled comedians can trigger empathy arising from the funny things that can happen to the unwary. Some television shows have portrayed such situations and raised awareness of life with such symptoms. For instance, in Australia the television series *Mother and Son* (1984–1994), with highly respected actors Gary McDonald and Ruth Cracknell, used this opportunity to provide an insightful social commentary on relationships affected by dementia symptoms. Other countries have similar shows, depicting confused or cognitively impaired people as eccentric or odd, such as the Double Dementia episode of United Kingdom BBC comedy 'The Visit' (BBC 2015). Other renderings include actor Will Ferral's representation of American president, Ronald Reagan with Alzheimer's disease (Spargo 2016).

Alternatively, the experience of having someone with dementia in a family can produce a stigmatising effect. Social stigma can be magnified by cultural attitudes that support misinformation and ageism, allowing spontaneous accusations of 'dementia' to be used to denigrate by suggesting that the target of the abuse is cognitively compromised. Such use of terminology by unqualified people can have the effect of undermining a person's self-confidence and spread doubts about the intellectual capacity of a person so labelled.

In recent decades researchers have commented on the misinformation that abounds among the general public about causes, symptoms and treatment of dementia-causing conditions. There is evidence of widespread ignorance about changes occurring in normal ageing, as well as dementia symptoms (see, for instance, Cahill *et al*. 2015; Neitch *et al*. 2016). This includes a general assumption, found in Australia and elsewhere, that all old people will eventually have dementia and become 'senile' if they live long enough. What is the link between these ideas?

The opportunity to care for someone with such symptoms provides a way to demonstrate one's humanity, loyalty, gratitude and tolerance. Those who live with dementia, or who provide care and support for them, are confronted with significant changes in relationships, roles and even personal aspirations. Without the largesse and loyalty of those around them, the future for a person with dementia is bleak indeed. A person who is befuddled and unable to be self-determining is at great risk of their personhood and identity being compromised. Despite one's life and achievements, and regardless of the intellectual contribution they may have made, upon receipt of a 'dementia' diagnosis, all that that person has been and done in life could be dismissed. If this occurs, others will then define the identity of the dementing person and make life-changing decisions for them. People labelled with a dementia 'diagnosis' can be placed in serviced accommodation and organised in ways that encourage routine conformity among those living there. The result is an artificially created sub-culture of people with cognitive deficit as their defining characteristic.

Efforts by regulators to make provision for those with dementia and to mandate standards for care and accommodation mitigate against highly routinised environments. Increasingly the rights of consumers of care to choose and direct services is being embedded in policies around government services (Mahoney *et al*. 2004; Low *et al*. 2012). However, the provision of dementia services is an expanding source of income for service providers, who receive government subsidies and benefits as well as charging service users for their products. Dementia research is also a plentiful source of grant funding for universities and research institutes; indeed, finding the 'cure' for dementia dominates the research agenda and has become the Holy Grail in biomedical research world-wide. The return on investment for companies that produce treatments or 'cures' for dementia symptoms will be substantial and economically justifies the focus of their interests.

Complicating social attitudes to dementia is inconsistency in medical understandings and practices. For example, advances in scientific understanding of dementia aetiology are not always understood or immediately adopted by clinicians in their assessment and treatment of dementia-like symptoms. The state of mental confusion may be due to biological or psychological factors and, depending on the underlying cause, may be reversible if accurately diagnosed and professionally treated (Mitchell *et al*. 2011). When diagnosing the cause of the symptoms, dementia should be weighed up against other possibilities.

Clinicians who fail to properly assess symptoms can make an unsubstantiated diagnosis of 'dementia' (Howard 2014). This not only consigns those so labelled to a future that will be plagued by untreated symptoms, they will also be subjected to the condescension of those who take over their decision-making. The only outcome that can be guaranteed by 'best guess' or a 'lazy' diagnosis of mental confusion is human misery. Under the United Nations Declaration of Human Rights, people are entitled to receive an evidence-based diagnosis and have access to appropriate treatment that protects their personal dignity and integrity.

Of the many thousands of people who are said to be living with dementia symptoms, many have been accurately diagnosed and treated. Two major studies in this area claim that level to be around 60 to 70 per cent (Matzo 1990; Mandingo and Middlemiss 1997). Temporary symptoms of confusion commonly manifest in older persons and, if diagnosed accurately and treated, are often reversible (McDonald 2009). However, treatment based on 'dementia' as an incorrect diagnosis has inherent risks of the symptoms remaining unresolved as well as the adverse effects of mistreatment (Narzarko 2006). For example, untreated chronic diseases can cause older adults to develop delirium, a temporary but dangerous condition caused by several factors that unskilled clinicians frequently diagnose as dementia. When the underlying condition remains untreated, and deteriorates, the person and family may doubt the value of wasting time attending medical appointments and paying out-of-pocket expenses that have no beneficial outcome. The consequences of misdiagnosis of, for example, Parkinson's disease, Creutzfeldt-Jacob disease, Huntingdon's chorea, Picks' disease and others, lies in the waste of time and expense on ineffective treatments for a condition they may not have (Mendez 2006).

The struggle to find dementia information that clarifies rather than bewilders is frustrating for the general population. Misinformation, ignorance, stereotyping, age discrimination and personal self-interest can influence attitudes and judgements made by family and friends as well as clinicians and service providers who disseminate such information. The absence of accurate and impartial information on dementia causation and treatment options has the potential to reduce the self-efficacy of people living with mental confusion, thereby increasing their vulnerability to criminal fraud, exploitation and abuse. The search for useful information is not helped by dramatic announcements from research institutes and other organisations of a 'tsunami of dementia' or an 'epidemic of dementia'. Such hyperbole strikes fear into the public and fortifies feelings of hopelessness and inevitability while enabling predators to target vulnerable adults.

## Competitive and abusive strategies as expressions of ageism

In a pragmatic sense, the emergence of a dementia-causing condition raises questions around mental capacity and the need to rely on others for legal, financial and often personal decision-making. In highly competitive, predatory families this can be an opportunity to strip assets from the afflicted person. For instance, if the owner of a property is declared mentally incompetent, the family member or friend who had the foresight to organise transfer of legal control at the moment of diagnosis could be in a position to make all future financial and other decisions about the person's wealth. They are not only in a position to control a person's assets but also to deny responsibility and distribution to others in the family. Of course, the nomination of such a person is designed to safeguard the interests of the person with dementia symptoms, and can be unproblematic in close and supportive families but there are ample examples of it dividing even these families. Within a society where ageism is normalised, people intent upon gaining control over another's resources can pervert systems and processes set up to support older people. An example of such a strategy is discussed below.

### Caring for mother

Mother, a recent widow, lives in the home she and her husband worked for decades to pay off and keep maintained while raising a family. Her son, daughter-in-law and two grandchildren move in with her to 'take care of her' in her grief. The children are noisy and destructive and the daughter-in-law unfriendly and lazy while the son ignores her. Social contact with her friends and other family is restricted by the unwelcoming attitudes of her son and daughter-in-law. The only time she has the house to 'herself' is at night when she sits in the unlit lounge room alone wondering what to do. After three months of having them there, she decides she has had enough and challenges her son about how she is being mistreated and asks him to take his family and leave her house. There is an argument and everyone is upset. That afternoon the son sees her general practitioner (GP) and expresses his deep concerns about her mental deterioration and tells a story of mother's irritability, possessiveness, forgetfulness, aggression towards the children and her wandering the house at night doing 'God-knows-what'. The GP comes to see her but she is so unhappy she cries and cannot clearly tell him what has happened. He diagnoses dementia and refers her for an aged care assessment team assessment for nursing home placement. Her distress at the possibility of being relocated to an aged care home is used by her son as further 'proof' that she has 'dementia' and the process continues as she sinks into deep depression and hopelessness.

In this scenario, the son has negatively positioned his mother's normal responses to being invaded, maltreated and eventually dispossessed of her home. Identity is based on the stories we tell about ourselves and when someone else takes over the telling of the stories and presents them in a negative way, our identity is re-shaped in the minds of others. The son's construction of events was endorsed by the GP, who subsequently influenced follow-up assessors to accept the son's narrative. By negatively repositioning her behaviour, the son and his family stripped her of the identity she had built up over her lifetime and will eventually strip her property away from her as well. Clinicians, service providers, legal representatives and regulators who are inclined to listen to the loudest, youngest voice or any narrative that confirms their own covert ageist prejudices, are complicit in exposing older people to abuse and exploitation.

Negative positioning can be used as justification in the predator's mind for the exploitation and abuse that they plan to undertake. This tactic has also been referred to as 'malignant positioning' (Sabat *et al.* 2009) when it occurs in the presence of cognitive deficit affecting the targeted person. When a person is said to 'have dementia' suddenly their world is forever changed. Anything one says following such a diagnosis can be dismissed as 'demented ramblings'; any displays of anger, frustration or despair classified as 'challenging behaviours'. Immediately their 'disposing memory' (a legal term referring to the mental competence of adults when writing a will or disposing of property) is questioned and family members or friends can take legal control of property and finances by convincing the relevant authorities that they are acting in the best interests of the compromised person. The strategy frequently used to achieve such an outcome is to negatively interpret the affected person's behaviour so that they are positioned within stereotypical narratives that undermine their personal integrity (Moghaddam *et al.* 2007).

Research on ageing and discrimination produces consistent evidence (see, for instance, MacNicol 2005; Cherubini *et al.* 2010; Kunze *et al.* 2011) that older people are treated differently and are subjected to covert discrimination around customs, practices and even exclusion from participation in research. The health and clinical consequences of this discrimination lie in older people with disabling mental disorders such as depression being less likely to be put in contact with health practitioners than younger people with similar problems. This disadvantage increases with age (Collier 2006). Ironically, Maynard (2003) found that, despite having disabling health problems, most older people rate themselves more highly on life satisfaction scales than family or health professionals do.

As one expression of ageism, depression is regarded as an expected outcome of being older and, therefore, unworthy of attention. Clinicians and others who harbour convictions that ageing will bring a decline in enthusiasm for life and involvement, will be more likely to use the convenient ageist diagnosis of 'dementia' instead of properly investigating the cause of symptoms. If ageist bigotry is tolerated as normal in a society, anyone aged over 60 risks becoming alienated, neglected or otherwise abused with impunity, a victim of crime that is regarded as socially acceptable.

The presence of dementia-causing illness can be used to promote interpersonal disconnection which in turn enables ageism, prejudice, bigotry, violence, fraud and neglect to be perpetrated on the afflicted person. In Australia the most common form of suspected abuse towards older adults is financial (theft and fraud) but it rarely occurs alone (McDonald and Greiner 2016). Usually it is thought to occur in tandem with neglect, social isolation and psychological abuse by middle-aged sons and daughters. When the goal of perpetrators is to derive financial benefit by removing an elderly parent from their debt-free home, for instance, a common strategy is to emotionally distress and then intellectually discredit them through negative positioning, with the help of clinicians and organisations deriving financial benefit from selling dementia services. In each step of this process there are opportunities for verifying the claims made and the bona fides of those seeking to access another's property. Until clinicians and managers are required to report such crimes and attacks there will be little to motivate them to act to protect older people and their property.

## Implications

Competition for resources within an individualistic society promotes 'winning at any cost' as an ideal. If one's competitors are less resourceful or capable, this provides a competitive advantage. Regulation in western societies is generally in place to ensure the preservation of human rights (United Nations 1948) as well as equitable access to society and community engagement. Recent regulatory responses to long-term atrocities against women and children have established prevention and intervention protocols with mandatory reporting to police and education of frontline workers to increase awareness of the signs of such activity. Currently in Australia there is no mandatory reporting of crimes and other abuses against older people, and despite the plight of those being exploited by their families or neglected by professional services, the issues have not been widely exposed to public scrutiny.

In western cultures adults are expected to be self-sufficient and there is a delineation between personal problems described in terms of personal responsibility and capacity to resolve them, and political problems relating to regulatory frameworks that identify inequities and move to safeguard those who are disadvantaged. Dementia is currently framed as a personal problem, therefore, the resources of that person or their family are expected to be used to resolve any issues. In the same way, a person's financial, health and social issues are considered personal and there is a reluctance by others external to the family to involve themselves in something that they consider to be 'none of their business'. The similarities in circumstance between domestic violence, child molesting and abuses of older people are obvious. In the former, a groundswell of public contempt for the perpetrators prompted regulators and police to act to protect the victims of these attacks – and this permitted others who became aware of attacks to get involved.

While similar public contempt and action is required in the case of abuse of older people, it can be anticipated that ageism as well as distorted understandings of dementia will make this more difficult. The process of raising awareness and proposing strategies for responding to breaches of human rights of older people begins with reframing 'dementia', from a medical and/or ageing issue to a political and social issue that is enabling abuses to occur. If public awareness is achieved, it becomes possible to focus policy attention on resourcing for capacity building of all involved.

Clearly, any competition for public attention and achieving shifts of public resources to a more empowering framework will be highly competitive. If successful, the focus of public investment would be moved from preserving the status quo, in which old people are marginalised within communities and some families, to a position where they have control over their own destiny and personal choices through active engagement as well as trustworthy and accountable advocates. Such shifts in power and control of resources will be confronting to those advantaged by current arrangements that allocate entrenched power to them and control of existing resources and messaging.

## The need for change

Healthy older adults, as well as those living with dementia symptoms, are being discriminated against and there is a need for society to acknowledge the damage caused by ageist stereotyping and how that enables exploitation. The marginalisation and alienation of older adults, especially those who have health issues, must stop. Only strong leadership can initiate this social change. Past infringements on the human rights of identifiable groups within western societies have prompted social movements that raise awareness and force action to be taken to identify those who profit from such maltreatment, or those whose policies enable atrocities against vulnerable individuals. Globally, we tried to achieve similar goals in the 1960 and 1970s with the Women's movement; we had greater success with the Disability Rights movement in the 1980s and 1990s; the Gay Rights movement has resulted in social awareness of homosexual issues; and more recently, the personal misery caused by the abuse of women and children in domestic contexts and the molestation of children by adults with power over them has been elevated to mainstream concern. It is time to raise public awareness of covert abuse and neglect of older adults, especially those with cognitive deficits, so that they can be welcomed and accepted by society rather than being disenfranchised on the basis of 'dementia' and alienated from their families and communities.

The urgent need for a movement against discrimination and victimisation of those with dementia lies in the effect that such bigotry will have on younger people 'pre-diagnosed' in their 30s and 40s, at a time when accurate diagnosis and effective treatment is either not available or not offered, and expensive for those who do access treatment. The stories of individual bravery by people with dementia symptoms against abuse, discrimination and bigotry will increase as younger people in their 40s, or younger, are pre-diagnosed with 'potential' Alzheimer's and, unlike older adults with such a label, they will face decades of discrimination unless we succeed in reframing dementia as a mainstream social concern for which options and solutions exist.

The fact that ageism and financial exploitation of older family members by their offspring is now widely normalised, means that it is time for this groundswell of resistance to occur. We need to raise the general understanding of normal changes associated with late age so that disease processes can clearly be identified and treated appropriately. Governments, businesses, clinicians and social leaders, including the media, are well positioned to lead the type of social change that has raised awareness of child abuse and domestic violence in recent times. It is important that we reframe elder abuse as the third part of a triptych of abuses occurring within trust relationships. It is only when society's leaders provide strong advocacy and are supported by community involvement, that understanding and effective interventions become possible. Such a unified campaign could end the widespread undermining of older adults' rights and security through negative positioning arising from prejudice or unfair competition for resources.

## References

Angus, J., P. Reeve, 2006, Ageism: A threat to 'aging well' in the 21st century, *Journal of applied gerontology*, 25(2): 137–152.

Atherden, G., 1984, *Mother and Son TV Series*, 1984–1994, www.imdb.com/title/tt0088573/ [Accessed 16 August 2017].

BBC Series, 2015, *The Visit: Double Dementia*, www.youtube.com/watch?v=MNUw2hFLRFk [Accessed 16 August 2017].

Burt, R.S., 1993, The social structure of competition, in Richard Swedberg (ed.), *Explorations in Economic Sociology*, pp. 65–103, New York: Russell Sage Foundation, J. Social Science.

Butler, R., 2005, Ageism: Looking back over my shoulder, *J. Generations, American Society on Aging*, 3: 84–86.

Cahill, S., M. Pierce, P. Werner, A. Darley, A. Bobersky, 2015, A systematic review of the public's knowledge and understanding of Alzheimer's Disease and dementia, *Alzheimer Disease and Associated Disorders*, 29(3): 255–275.

Cherubini, A., S. Del Signore, J. Ouslander, T. Semla, J.P. Michel, 2010, Fighting against age discrimination in clinical trials, *Journal of American Geriatrics Society*, 58(9): 1791–1796.

Collier, E., 2006, Mental health and functional disorder in older adults, *J. Nursing Elder People*, 18(9): 25–32.

Howard, R., 2014, Doubts about dementia diagnoses, *The Lancet*, 4(8): 580–581.

Kunze, F., S.A. Boehm, H. Bruch, 2011, Age diversity, age discrimination climate and performance consequences: A cross organizational study, *Journal of Organizational Behavior*, 32(2): 264–290.

Low, L.F., N. Chilko, M. Gresham, S. Barter, H. Brodaty, 2012, An update on the pilot trial of consumer-directed care for older persons in Australia, *Australasian Journal on Ageing*, 31(1): 47–50.

MacNicol, J., 2005, *Age Discrimination: An Historical and Contemporary Analysis*, Cambridge, UK: Cambridge University Press.

Mahoney, K.J., L. Simon-Rusinowitz, D. Loughlin, S.M. Desmond, M.R. Squillace, 2004, Determining personal care consumers' preferences for a consumer-directed cash and counselling option: Survey results from Arkansas, Florida, New Jersey, and New York elders and adults with physical disabilities, *Health Services Research*, 39(3): 643–664.

Mandingo, M., C. Middlemiss, 1997, Alzheimer's disease: Preventing and recognizing misdiagnosis, *The Nurse Practitioner*, 22(10): 58–75.

Matzo, M., 1990, Confusion in older adults: Assessment and differential diagnosis, *The Nurse Practitioner*, 15(9): 32–46.

Maynard, C.K., 2003, Differentiate depression from dementia, *The Nurse Practitioner*, 28(3): 18–27.

Mcadams, D.P., 2006, The problem of narrative coherence, *Journal of Constructivist Psychology*, 19(2): 109–125.

McDonald, T., 2012, Elemental considerations of long life as success or failure, *Journal of Religion, Spirituality and Aging*, 24: 1–2, 4–19.

McDonald, T., 2009, Dementia is a symptom, not a definitive diagnosis, *International Association of Homes and Services for the Ageing (IAHSA) 8th International Conference*, London 20–22 July 2009.

McDonald, T., K. Greiner, 2016, Combating ageism: A challenge for all ages and all sectors, *International Federation on Ageing 13th Global Conference*, Brisbane, Australia 21–23 June 2016.

Mendez, M., 2006, The accurate diagnosis of early-onset dementia, *International Journal of Psychiatry and Medicine*, 36(4): 401–412.

Miller D.T., 1999, The norm of self-interest, *American Psychological Association*, 54(12): 1053–1060.

Miskimmon, R.A., B. O'Loughlin, 2014, Strategic narrative: A new means to understand soft power, *Media, War & Conflict*, 7(1): 70–84.

Mitchell A.J., N. Meader, M. Pentzek, 2011, Clinical recognition of dementia and cognitive impairment in primary care: A meta-analysis of physician accuracy, *Acta Psychiatrica Scandanavia*, 124(3): 165–183.

Moghaddam, F.M., R. Harré, N. Lee (eds), 2007, *Global Conflict Resolution Through Positioning Analysis*, New York: Springer Science and Business Media, LLC.

Narzarko, L., 2006, Recognising the signs and symptoms of dementia, *Nursing and Residential Care Journal*, 8(1): 32–34.

Neitch, S.M., C. Meadows, E. Patton-Tackett, K.W. Yingling, 2016, Dementia care: Confronting myths in clinical management, *West Virginia Medical Journal*, 112(2): 32–36.

Sabat, S.R., R. Harré, F.M. Moghaddam, T. Pilkerton Cairnie, D. Rothbart, 2009, Recent advances in positioning theory, *Journal of Theory and Psychology*, 19(1): 5–31.

Schwartz, B., 1986, *The Battle for Human Nature*, New York: Norton.

Spargo, C., 2016, Will Ferrell pulls out of comedy about Ronald Reagan's battle with Alzheimer's one day after former president's children attack actor for taking on role, *Daily Mail*, www.dailymail.co.uk/news/article-3566143/Will-Ferrell-pulls-comedy-Ronald-Reagan-s-battle-Alzheimer-s-one-day-former-president-s-children-attack-actor-taking-role.html [Accessed 16 August 2017].

United Nations, 1948, *Universal Declaration of Human Rights*, as adopted by the United Nations General Assembly on 10 December 1948, Paris, France.

# 3 'Nobody cares about me'

## Older women, caring and dementia

*Jane Mears*

## Gender and care

In an increasingly unequal and discriminatory society, in which ageism, sexism and racism have been exacerbated, older women face a precarious future. My task in this chapter is to make these women more visible, especially in the context of living with dementia. My aim is to not simply highlight the precarity of their lives, and to show that investing in care will generate significant social and economic benefits, but also to recognise what we have to learn from these women, who not only carry a great weight of care, under untenable conditions, but have been doing this work for decades, demonstrating astonishing dignity, courage and commitment.

In this chapter I look at gender and care and the ways in which care is gendered, particularly care for those living with dementia, the economics of care, the centrality of care to all our lives and finally, what we can learn about care and caring from older women, particularly in the context of caring for and about those living with dementia.

Care is a gendered activity. Women carry the bulk of the responsibility for those needing care: children, those with disabilities and older people. Across the globe, about two-thirds of informal care for frail older people falls to women (Andrews 2016). Caring is, for many women, a part of life that is taken for granted, with the provision of informal care deeply embedded within the everyday responsibilities and duties of family life.

Caring is invisible. In the United Kingdom, it was found that of the 4511 people surveyed, more than half (51 per cent) believed they do not know a single family member or friend who cares, whilst as many as three in five workers (62 per cent) believed they do not know 'any work colleagues' who help look after a loved one. In reality, one in ten (10 per cent) people in the United Kingdom are carers and one in nine people in the workforce are juggling their paid jobs with unpaid caring (Carers UK 2017).

Caring work is viewed as lower status than work outside the home and is usually allocated to women. Even in societies where there is support for gender equality, men earn more than women, and it is most often women who give up paid work to care (Andrews 2016).

Across the world, most of the care needed by older people, be they frail, sick or disabled, is provided with no pay or remuneration, by unpaid informal care givers, within the family. In Australia, 90 per cent of care for older people and those with disability, is provided by informal carers, family and friends. Indeed, there are over 2,646,020 informal carers (ABS 2016). This is likely to be an underestimate, as people providing support, help and assistance to family members or friends may not actually identify themselves as a 'carer' (Cass and Yeandle 2009).

Women are mostly willing carers, even though most do not really have a choice. They take on caring with little recognition or support. However, there are significant financial, health and emotional costs of caring. Many carers suffer adverse health impacts as a result of caring; they are at a greater risk of negative physical and mental health effects. Those who provide high levels of intensive care are even more vulnerable (Australian Human Rights Commission 2013).

## Gender and dementia care

Older women make up the majority of those caring for people with dementia, both as informal carers and as paid care workers in home care and residential aged care. Between 60 per cent and 70 per cent of informal carers of those with dementia are women. Carers of people with dementia tend to provide more intensive and extensive care than carers of people with other conditions, and caring for someone with dementia is known to be more demanding and stressful than caring for people who are physically impaired (Brodaty *et al.* 2005).

Surveys of informal carers for people with dementia indicate there are 2.5-times more women than men who provide intensive, 24 hour a day care for someone with dementia (Alzheimer's Research UK 2015). Women are likely to delay placement of a family member in residential care, even at the expense of their own health and wellbeing (Bamford and Walker 2012). Women who care for people with dementia also feel less supported than their male counterparts. Wives caring for their husbands with severe dementia reported receiving less support from friends and family than husbands caring for their wives in similar circumstances (Alzheimer's Research UK 2015). Caregivers of people with dementia have lower levels of life satisfaction and higher levels of anxiety and depression than caregivers in any other context (Brodaty *et al.* 2005).

Also, when older women find themselves the carers of those with dementia, their futures become even more precarious, socially and economically. Women are more likely to reduce their hours or stop working to care for someone with dementia, and often feel penalised at work for taking on care responsibilities. In the United Kingdom, nearly 19 per cent of women who care for someone with dementia have had to quit work, either to become a carer or because their care-giving duties became a priority. Among working women carers, 20 per cent have gone from working full time to part time, compared with only 3 per cent of working male carers (Alzheimer's Research UK 2015).

As if this was not burden enough, older women are disproportionately impacted by dementia. It is estimated that 61 per cent of people with dementia worldwide are women, while 39 per cent are men (Alzheimer's Research UK 2015). In Australia women are the majority of those with dementia living in residential aged care (Australian Institute of Health and Welfare 2012).

Bamford and Walker (2012) described these older women living with dementia, as facing a 'triple jeopardy' as a consequence of the stigma attached to their age, gender and dementia.

Despite decades of work on the gender implications of caring and informal care, it is only recently that researchers have started to pay attention to the disproportionate impact of dementia on older women. Gender is rarely mentioned in public discourse relating to those living with dementia. Even though women are the most impacted on by dementia, and caring for and about those with dementia, in most of the research papers, reports and policies there is no mention of gender as a risk factor for dementia, and no distinction made between men and women.

In their review of research on dementia, Bartlett and colleagues (2016) found that most of the studies they looked at did not consider gender differences. The studies focused on (degendered) informal carers, with no mention of gender in the context of those with dementia. As such, questions about gender equality are not being raised and the voices of men and women with dementia are silent. In addition, because a dementia diagnosis tends to exclude people from mainstream ageing studies, little attention has been paid to older women with dementia even within areas of feminist enquiry. This is a significant oversight: we need a critical feminism for people with dementia too (Bartlett *et al.* 2016).

Women are invisible in the National Dementia strategies of countries such as Australia, Denmark, Finland, France, Israel, Republic of Korea, Luxembourg, Malta, The Netherlands, Norway, Northern Ireland, Switzerland, Taiwan, United Kingdom and United States. In a report by Alzheimer's International (2017), although there is a suggestion that 'Perhaps the most vital component of any dementia plan is the inclusion of people with dementia in both the policy and implementation processes', there is no mention made at all of women or gender inequality.

However, gender, as well as age, is an important factor structuring the lives of those living with dementia (Bartlett *et al.* 2016). There are gender differences in the caregiving experience and 'gender clearly matters in the context of illness, impairment and care-giving' (Annandale and Hunt 2000). Milligan and Thomas point out that, for example,

> if you have middle stage dementia and are female, old and poor you may be more vulnerable to aspects of disablism and other faces of oppression (sexism, ageism etc.) than if you have middle stage dementia but are male ... old and from a professional background.

> (2016)

It is especially important with respect to people with a disability like dementia where 'forms and impacts of disablism are always refracted in some way through the prism of gendered locations and gender relations' (Thomas 1999: 28). For example, the loss of a handbag is thought to symbolise the loss of independence for a woman with dementia (Buse and Twigg 2014); and a man with dementia in a care home may feel socially excluded because there are few other men to relate to (Bartlett and O'Connor 2007).

The slippage between rhetoric and action impacts disproportionately on older women. In fact, there is a contradiction: what does it mean to acknowledge and embrace the important contribution of those caring for people with dementia, when the majority of these carers are women? These women experience so much discrimination even before they face the challenges of dementia, with dementia themselves or as carers for those with dementia. These older women experience a complex form of hardship: they not only have to deal with the isolation and lack of support experienced by carers of those with dementia, they are also marginalised and socially excluded because of ageism and sexism.

## The economics of care

The exploitative nature of care expectations is evident in the economics of care. The economic value of unpaid care to the economy is huge, however, the personal costs carried by women are very high.

Carers Australia estimate that informal care in Australia 'saves' the economy a massive $60.3 billion. Informal carers contribute about 1.9 billion hours of unpaid care. This is equivalent to each carer providing 673 hours per year or 13 hours per week. If all hours of informal care provided in 2015 are replaced with services purchased from formal care providers, the replacement value of informal care would be the aforementioned $60.3 billion, which is equivalent to 3.8 per cent of gross domestic product and 60 per cent of the health and social work industry (Carers Australia 2015).

The undervaluing of women's contributions to unpaid care has a significant impact on women's retirement income and savings. Many Australian women face an insecure retirement. Men's superannuation balances at retirement are on average twice as large as women's. In practice this means that women, particularly single women, are at greater risk of experiencing poverty, housing stress and homelessness in retirement.

This is a problem born of many interrelated factors. At its heart, however, is the fact that women and men experience work very differently. Women are more likely to work in lower paid roles and lower paid fields, are more likely to work part-time or casually and are more likely to take breaks from paid employment to provide unpaid care for others. Over their lifetimes, as a consequence, women will earn significantly less than men.

Given the high proportion of care undertaken by women the undervaluing of unpaid care work has had the greatest impact in economic terms on women's retirement incomes and savings. In 2009–2010, the average (mean) superannuation balance for all men was $71,645, whereas the comparable figure for all women was $40,475.4 (Australian Human Rights Commission 2013).

## Care is integral to human social life

The demand for care services far outstrips the supply of services. Ironically, Australia has a good coverage of home care services, with over one million Australians receiving government subsidised care in their homes. However, these services are spread very sparsely, with the overwhelming majority of older people receiving only a few hours of support per week. In 2016, 925,000 older people received on average, two hours of home care a week. Most of these people were happy with the support they received, but most reported needing more help. Two hours assistance per week does not go very far. Only 89,000 people were receiving the more intensive home care support. In addition, 57,000 received residential respite care and there were 235,000 people in permanent residential aged care (Commonwealth of Australia 2017: 39).

In addition, finding out about services is difficult and even once you have been assessed as eligible, the waiting lists, and thus the waiting times, are very long. In September 2017 it was reported that nearly 90,000 Australians approved for the Home Care Packages Program were unable to access the care they needed: 53,000 were waiting for a package, while 35,000 were making do with less care than they needed. A further 67,000 were waiting to be transferred to a higher-level package, so they could receive more hours (Belardi 2017). The number in this 'national queue' grew by 14.2 per cent from 30 June 2017 to 30 September 2017 (Bolden 2017), and in early 2018 was at over 100,000, with an average waiting time of 18 months.

While people are waiting for care, they either miss out altogether, or care continues to be is provided by, often overloaded and very stressed, informal carers. We do not know how many of these are waiting for care in the context of dementia, but their care needs are arguably more intense than for any other kind of care. It is hardly surprising that there is little expectation that people with dementia can be cared for at home: carers are insufficiently supported to do so.

Those with dementia want accessible, affordable, supportive, sensitive and compassionate care in their own homes, with the choice to access palliative care and high quality residential care when needed. This should not sound like a 'wish list' but it is. We know what is needed, and how to deliver it.

What is getting in the way? In this section I want to address the social values and assumptions underpinning policies and programmes that currently stand in the way of us achieving a caring society, as well as what is needed as we work for change.

The context of reforms to long-term care globally is shaped by neoliberalism and the impact of what is known as 'new public management' (NPM) on the development of long-term care systems worldwide. NPM was an attempt to improve the public service through the use of private sector efficiency models, and has led to the marketisation of care. The expansion of long-term care thus occurred at a time when new public management had had considerable influence on policy development internationally. In Australia, the influence of this management approach could be seen on reforms to long-term care from the 1980s, with progressive waves of reform moving towards greater national regulation and increasing marketisation and competition. Throughout this period there have been constant underlying tensions between providing high quality support and services for older people, demonstrating quantifiable outcomes and balancing budgets (Mears 2018).

However, care is about relationships and caring for all, not just those who can afford to pay. The marketisation and the privatisation of care means that, in general, those who receive most care are the ones who have the greatest resources; those with fewer resources receive less care. The 'austerity measures' that wealthier, most often western, nations enacted as a response to the global economic crisis entailed cuts in care services and in welfare entitlements impacting on the most marginalised and vulnerable people (Branelly *et al.* 2017: 9).

The implication is, of course, that care is integral to human social life and cannot be defined as a 'cost' or societal burden in the way some would like us to believe. It can be argued that those who work are caring for those who do not, but this argument rests on an understanding that life is social, and that it is not about maximising the benefits of individuals at the expense of others.

Care takes place within a societal system of relationship and obligation. It is fundamental to all human life, not a burden nor an option. Care has to be a social value not just a task, albeit one that falls mostly on women. It is not only those who are ill or vulnerable who require care, so too do carers. Who is caring for those who support those with dementia? The carer is, and ultimately, the society. It is the society that must ensure that its own are looked after from birth to death. The responsibility for care is everyone's, and it is when care is demeaned by contrasting it to the 'usefulness' of 'work' that a host of discriminations work to exclude and marginalise this vulnerable group. As one carer told me, 'Nobody cares about me. I actually see this lack of support for carers as a sign of an uncaring society'.

Structural and cultural violence are forms of violence in which social structures, social institutions and social arrangements, and the cultural ideologies that sustain and reproduce these, serve to marginalise and exclude certain categories of people (Galtung 1969, 1990). The social values and practices that encourage ageism and sexism manifest in discrimination against individuals or groups on the basis of their age and gender.

Structural discrimination, in areas such as care, care services, education and employment, are also exacerbated by the intersection of age, gender and cumulative disadvantage, particularly for older women (Australian Council of Social Services 2015). Structural violence impacts dramatically on the full realisation of the human rights of older women (Choi *et al.* 2015). We need to identify and address both the cultural ideas that legitimises these structural inequities, as well as change the structures through which they find expression, if we are to improve the lives of older women. Given their role as carers, this will also improve the quality of care they are able to deliver.

We are already facing a crisis of care, particularly the provision of social- and relationship-based care for those with dementia. This impacts on us all. We are living in an era where critiques of marketisation have become obscured and 'responsibility' has become an individual obligation, rather than the collective responsibilities of citizens and states. The claim of those with dementia for a right to relationship-based, flexible and individualised care, like other claims for rights, is made within the liberal paradigm and, the call of the disability rights movement for justice, rights and self-determination has been readily absorbed into liberal discourses, rather than fundamentally challenging the structural impediments (Branelly *et al.* 2017).

Tronto (2017) argues that care has the potential to interrogate relationships of power to reveal how current institutional arrangements support inequality and injustice. This is the critical approach needed to enact a paradigm shift, one that moves from understanding that many of the problems experienced by older women are not the problems of individuals but are socially-constituted; and that understands care as a societal responsibility. Drawing on critical gender theory, she argues for the reclaiming of a critical agenda based on anti-ageist challenges from the Carers' Movement and disability activists, as well as critical research into the co-creation and co-production of person-centred care (Tronto 2017).

This care paradigm stands in stark contradiction to the dominant discourse, which is positioning caring as a private responsibility, which should be provided by the family or (increasingly) the market. Neoliberal economic and political policies downplay citizenship and society, and thus the notion of the social good or the common weal. In this context, improvements to policy and practices around care become a perennial struggle. The value distinction between those who work/produce and/or are financially independent, and those who are 'dependent' or a burden on the society, is a product of neoliberal ideas. In privileging a certain kind of entrepreneurial self as a 'norm' (Dardot and Laval 2013), these economised values create discriminations that, in the mid-twentieth century, we thought we were moving beyond: sexism, racism and ageism in particular. Neoliberal, masculinist values are driving economic and political decision-making at the expense of values of care, women and those being cared for, especially older women.

## Paid care workers

We see the repercussions of this in cost cutting, i.e. the low pay of workers in aged care services. This also impacts dramatically on older women. In Australia, around 10 per cent of the care and support provided to older people, is provided through formal (government subsidised) long-term care services, by paid care workers, in home care and residential care homes. Women make up the majority of the paid workforce, in home care (89 per cent) and in residential aged care (87 per cent). These women are older workers, with a median age of 52 years in home care and 46 years in residential aged care (Mavromaras *et al.* 2017). Indeed, aged care, home care and residential care were the second most common industries for employed older women in 2016 (Australian Bureau of Statistics 2017).

Most of this care is provided to older people in the home and in residential care facilities, behind closed doors. Paid care work, like informal care work is invisible, taken for granted and given little status and accorded little value. Evesson and Oxenbridge report that

> care workers experience deep frustration stemming from: their 'invisible' status; a lack of respect from managers and the wider society for the professional, skilled and complex work they perform; and management assumptions that they do this work not to earn a living but 'for love'.
>
> (2017: 7)

The financial remuneration for care workers is abysmal, with low pay rates seen by care workers' as further evidence that their work is undervalued and, combined with insufficient work hours, causing severe financial stress (Evesson and Oxenbridge 2017). Nevertheless, the quality of care workers strive to provide is often high and most care workers reported that they frequently work over and above their allocated hours in order to give the care they judge is needed (Mears 2009).

In addition, there are few opportunities for promotion, a paucity of training opportunities, no formal training or educational level required in many jobs and little formal recognition of prior knowledge or experience, paid or unpaid (Mears 2009: 147).

At the very time when the need and demand for care in the home is increasing, with the ageing of the population, with people living longer lives and a predicted shortfall of informal carers as increasing numbers of women are in paid employment, the number of home care workers is declining. In 2016 there were 366,000 care workers in the aged care sector, 130,000 in home care 236,000 in residential aged care. However, in 2012 there had been approximately 150,000 home care workers. The decline is even greater when measured in terms of full-time equivalent staff, with 'a 19 per cent fall in the home care and home support full-time equivalent carer workforce'. This amounted to 10,450 less workers, from 54,537 in 2012 to 44,087 in 2016. This represents a further erosion of employment conditions of care workers. Fewer care workers work full time and those working are required to do more (Commonwealth of Australia 2017: 175).

## Learning from older women

Although this is a depressing scenario, there are millions of informal carers working at the coalface, who understand and 'get' these structural constraints and contest these ideas. What does it mean to acknowledge and embrace the important contribution of those caring for people with dementia when the majority of these carers are women and women experience so much discrimination even before they face the challenges of dementia, with dementia themselves or as carers for those with dementia? These older women experience a complex form of hardship: they not only have to deal with the isolation and lack of support experienced by carers of those with dementia, they are also marginalised and socially excluded because of ageism and sexism. It is evident that ageism and sexism contribute to Australia's failure to recognise, particularly in economic terms, both the worth and impact of unpaid caring roles. We need to recognise this caring, and alongside this recognise that these older women are carrying an unsustainable load.

Informal carers, and organisations representing informal carers have been active and vocal for almost five decades, persistently representing the interests and voices of informal carers and telling us this story, pushing for recognition and support. The work done by carers' associations, initiated, managed and run by informal carers, provide a solid foundation for building an understanding of older women's experiences of caring for those with dementia. An understanding of these experiences can assist us in rethinking, reframing and deepening analyses of gendered care that can challenge the sexist and ageist paradigms that underpin women's experiences of caring, and their precarity.

Carers associations have worked strategically alongside, and formed strong alliances with organisations representing older people, trade unions, nurses and care workers, care providers and other special interest groups. Many of these advocacy organisations are led by experienced older women. These women, born in the late 1940s and early 1950s, lived through the protests of the 1960s and 1970s, and benefitted from the opening up of higher education in the 1970s. They have been working as community activists and fighting gender-based inequality all their lives. They are now growing older, and have personal experience of the long-term impact of the combination of sexism and ageism on older women. The personal is once again becoming political and they are now advocating alongside and on behalf of, all older women.

These advocacy groups have decades of experience in bringing hidden stories, the stories of informal carers, of paid care workers and older women into the public domain, putting caring firmly on the public agenda. One of the first published accounts that directed attention to the complexity and importance of informal care was an excellent report by Stevenson (1975), titled *Dedication*. Stevenson, a carer herself, was President of Carers New South Wales when she wrote this report. Since that time, there have been many volumes of commissioned and partnered reports and research projects, and advocacy groups have made numerous submissions to government inquiries, providing up-to-date research, knowledge and understanding that has effectively kept caring on the social, political and research agenda.

These groups share similar visions and goals. They are calling for a sustainable aged care system, that provides high quality care for all older Australians, care that is flexible, relationship based, compassionate and reliable, both in the home and in residential aged care.

The arguments are straightforward. Informal carers need home care workers to provide support and sustain the caring enterprise, particularly for those caring for people with dementia. They want to be supported in the care they are providing, and also, to be supported in regard to their choices, about the amount and intensity of the care they are able to be provide. Many are wanting (and needing) to remain in paid work, and ensure their own future independence.

We all want to be able to care and be well cared for as we age. We want a supportive sustainable system of long-term care where we can access care when we need it. Most of us want to be cared for in our own homes, and indeed most of us want to die in our own homes. We want care that is individually tailored to our needs, is respectful, compassionate and relationship based. None of us want to be treated badly, marginalised and excluded from our families, friends and communities. Most of us would also like to be supported by community care, with well qualified professional care workers assisting us, with help with intimate tasks, such as bathing and heavy tasks, such washing, shopping and cleaning.

If we are to create a sustainable system of aged care and a caring society, we need to invest in the care workforce. Otherwise, with continued population ageing, and moves towards greater marketisation and privatisation of care, existing inequalities will be exacerbated. This will leave many vulnerable people – mostly older women who have cared all their lives and have few resources – with no one to care for them. We need to invest in home care services and increase substantially the numbers of aged care workers, improve remuneration and employment and working conditions, provide training and higher education opportunities and opportunities for promotion and career development. We need a skilled and well-resourced workforce, to support those living with dementia.

## Conclusion

To create a sustainable, high quality system of long-term care in Australia, it is absolutely imperative that we place issues of concern to older women at the forefront of public debate and policy development and advocate for structural changes to alleviate social inequality and include and support older women. We can also mount a powerful case for a fair share of resources to be allocated to older women to redress past injustices suffered by older women.

The desires and interests of those needing care, informal carers and paid care workers are very closely aligned. All of us working and living with dementia want acknowledgement and support. Many older women want to be able to make the very basic choice of whether or not to take on major caring responsibilities. None of us want to care simply because no one else is going to do it. Those of us who choose to care, want our work acknowledged and we want to be well supported in our care work and to be able to choose to continue with paid work if we want and/or need to.

This requires all of us, working together, for change to make the world a better place for all older people, a world where older women with dementia and working with those with dementia, are respected, nurtured and included. Dementia is not a personal problem, it is not just the concern of older women, dementia is everybody's business.

## References

Australian Bureau of Statistics (ABS), 2016, *A Profile of Carers, In Australia 4430.0 – Disability, Ageing and Carers, Australia: Summary of Findings, 2015*, www.abs.gov. au/ausstats/abs@.nsf/Latestproducts/4430.0Mainpercent20Features602015?opendocu ment&tabname=Summary&prodno=4430.0&issue=2015&num=&view= [Accessed 15 March 2018].

ABS, 2017, *Ageing in Australia 2071.0 – Census of Population and Housing: Reflecting Australia - Stories from the Census, 2016*, www.abs.gov.au/ausstats/abs@.nsf/Lookup/ by%20Subject/2071.0~2016~Main%20Features~Ageing%20Population~14 [Accessed 15 March 2018]

Alzheimer's International, 2017, *Alzheimer's International 2017, National Plans Examples 2017*, www.alz.co.uk/sites/default/files/pdfs/national-plans-examples-2017. pdf [Accessed 18 March 2018].

Alzheimer's Research UK, 2015, *Women and Dementia: A Marginalised Majority*, www. alzheimersresearchuk.org/wp-content/uploads/2015/03/Women-and-Dementia-A-Marginalised-Majority1.pdf [Accessed 20 October 2017].

Annandale, E., K. Hunt, 2000, *Gender Inequalities in Health*, Open University Press, www.mheducation.co.uk/openup/chapters/0335203647.pdf [Accessed 18 March 2018].

Andrews, J., 2016, The ageing population is a threat to women's economic welfare, *The Conversation*, 13 April 2016, https://theconversation.com/the-ageing-population-is-a-threat-to-womens-economic-welfare-57288 [Accessed 18 March 2018].

Australian Council of Social Services, 2015, *Inequality in Australia: A Nation Divided*, Australian Council of Social Services, www.acoss.org.au/wp content/uploads/2015/06/ Inequality_in_Australia_FINAL.pdf [Accessed 20 October 2017].

Australian Human Rights Commission, 2013, *Investing in Care: Recognising and Valuing Those Who Care*, Volume 1: Research Report, Sydney: Australian Human Rights Commission.

Australian Institute of Health and Welfare (AIHW), 2012, *Dementia in Australia*, www. aihw.gov.au/getmedia/199796bc-34bf-4c49-a046-7e83c24968f1/13995.pdf.aspx?inline =true [Accessed 18 March 2018].

Bamford, S., T. Walker, 2012, Women and dementia – Not forgotten, *Maturitas*, 73: 121–126.

Bartlett, R., D. O'Connor, 2007, From personhood to citizenship: Broadening the lens for dementia practice and research, *Journal of Aging Studies*, 21: 107–118

Bartlett, R., T. Gjernes, A. Lotherington, A. Obstefelder, 2016, Gender, citizenship and dementia care: A scoping review of studies to inform policy and future research, *Health and Social Care in the Community*, 23(1): 14–26.

Belardi, L., 2017, Home care data reveals 90,000 package shortfall, *Community Care Review*, 15 September 2017, www.australianageingagenda.com.au/2017/09/15/home-care-data-reveals-90000-package-shortfall/ [Accessed 18 March 2018].

Bolden, S., 2017, Home care packages waiting list grows by 14%, *iCare Health Blog*, 17 December 2017, www.icarehealth.com.au/blog/home-care-packages-waiting-list-grows-by-14/ [Accessed 17 March 2018].

Brannelly, T., M. Barnes, L. Ward (eds), 2017, *Ethics of Care: Critical Advances in International Perspective*, Bristol, UK: Policy Press.

Brodaty, H., C. Thompson, M. Fine, 2005, Why caregivers of people with dementia and memory loss don't use services, *International Journal of Geriatric Psychiatry*, 20: 537–546.

Buse, C.E., J.M. Twigg, 2014, Women with dementia and their handbags: Negotiating identity, privacy and 'home' through material culture, *Journal of Aging Studies*, 30: 14–22.

Carers Australia, 2015, *The Economic Value of Informal Care in Australia in 2015*, http://www.carersaustralia.com.au/storage/Access%20Economics%20Report.pdf [Accessed 05 May 2018].

Carers UK, 2017, *Make Connections, Get Support: Recognising ourselves and other as carers*, www.carersuk.org/for-professionals/policy/policy-library/make-connections-get-support [Accessed 18 March 2018].

Cass, B., S. Yeandle, 2009, Policies for carers in Australia and the UK, social policy ideas, practices and their cross-national transmission: Social movements, parliamentary inquiries and local innovations, *RC19*, http://www.cccg.umontreal.ca/rc19/PDF/Cass-B_Rc192009.pdf [Accessed 05 May 2018].

Choi, M., P. Brownell, S. Moldovan, 2015, International movement to promote human rights of older women with a focus on violence and abuse against older women, *International Social Work*, 1–12.

Commonwealth of Australia, 2017, *Legislated Review of Aged Care 2017*, https://agedcare.health.gov.au/reform/aged-care-legislated-review [Accessed 05 May 2018].

Dardot, P., C. Laval, 2013, *The New Way of the World: On Neoliberal Society*, New York: Verso Books.

Evesson, J., S. Oxenbridge, 2017, *The Psychosocial Health and Safety of Australian Home Care Workers: Risks and Solutions*, Canberra, Australia: Employment Research Australia.

Galtung, J., 1969, Violence peace and peace research, *Journal of Peace Research*, 6(3): 167–191.

Galtung, J., 1990, Cultural violence, *Journal of Peace Research*, 27(3): 291–305.

Mears, J., 2009, Blurred boundaries: How paid careworkers and care managers negotiate work relationships, in D. King, D. and G. Meagher (eds), *Paid Care in Australia: Politics, Profits, Practices*, pp. 145–166, Sydney: Sydney University Press.

Mears, J., 2018, Reforms to long-term care in Australia: A changing and challenging landscape, in K. Christensen and D. Pilling, (eds), *A Handbook of Social Care Research: Care Work Research Around the World*, pp. 303–316, Farnham, UK: Ashgate.

Mavromaras, K., G. Knight, L. Isherwood, A. Crettenden, J. Flavel, T. Karmel, M. Moskos, M.L. Smith, H. Walton, Z. Wei, 2017, *The Aged Care Workforce, 2016*, Canberra: Australian Government Department of Health, https://agedcare.health.gov.au/sites/g/files/net1426/f/documents/03_2017/nacwcs_final_report_290317.pdf [Accessed 28 June 2017].

Milligan, C., C. Thomas, 2016, Dementia and the social model of disability: Does responsibility to adjust lie with society rather than people with dementia?, http://eprints.lancs.ac.uk/80176/1/SignpostArticle2.pdf [Accessed 20 October 2017].

Stevenson, C., 1975, *Dedication: A Report of a Survey on Caring for the Aged at Home*, Sydney: NSW Council on the Ageing.

Thomas, C., 1999, *Female Forms: Experiencing and Understanding Disability*, Buckingham, UK: Open University Press.

Tronto, J., 2017, Democratic caring and global care responsibilities, in T. Brannelly, and M. Barnes, L. Ward (eds), *Ethics of Care: Critical Advances in International Perspective*, pp. 21–30, Bristol, UK: Policy Press.

# 4 Feeling invisible and ignored

## Families' experiences of marginalisation living with younger onset dementia

*Karen Hutchinson, Chris Roberts and Pamela Roach*

### Introduction

This chapter reports on a research study that explored the impact of living with younger onset dementia (YOD) on both self and family members, including children and young people, from the perspective of the social model of disability. Through excerpts from interviews with people living with YOD, their partners, their children and lone children caring for parents with dementia, we illustrate their social isolation and discrimination. All the participants in our study spoke of feeling invisible and ignored, demonstrating poignantly, the powerful impact of societal marginalisation on those living with dementia, including their families, and ultimately, communities. By using the lens of the social model of disability, our study reframed living with dementia from a personal medical tragedy to a social issue which affects whole families. Such a shift in community perceptions could help bring about a social change that supports enablement and inclusion in society for all those impacted by dementia. Taking this social approach demands that support and services should be designed and developed collaboratively with impacted families, to ensure their rights to receiving timely age-appropriate care and support is achieved and becomes the norm.

Living with YOD has been described as 'contextually different' to that of living with the more prevalent late-onset dementia (LOD) (Spreadbury and Kipps 2017: 2). It is known to bring extra challenges for those of working age. This includes greater financial obligations, addressing the fact that there are more likely to be dependent children and young adults living at home (Brodaty and Donkin 2009; Gelman and Greer 2011) who will require specially tailored support services. However, it seems that levels of support and services to individuals and families living with YOD have been impacted by the problem of determining the global prevalence of YOD (Lambert *et al.* 2014). Accordingly, there has been little change in services for people living with YOD and their caregivers over the last three decades, even with an increase in the diagnosis of YOD worldwide (Mayrhofer *et al.* 2017). This is socially significant, and the needs of families living with YOD have gone largely unnoticed over this period of time. The lack of development in age-appropriate support and services not only impacts the lives of people living with YOD but all their family members, including children and young people (Allen *et al.* 2009; Van Vliet *et al.* 2010b; Svanberg *et al.* 2011; Johannessen and Moller 2013; Barca *et al.* 2014; Hall and Sikes 2016; Hutchinson *et al.* 2016b; Johannessen *et al.* 2016). Despite these issues, there have been few studies that have focused on the range of support services required to address the needs of the family as a whole, over the trajectory of living with YOD (Van Vliet *et al.* 2010b; Gelman and Greer 2011; Roach *et al.* 2014).

Much of the research related to individuals and families living with YOD emphasises family dysfunction, social isolation and unmet support and service needs for the whole family (Roach *et al.* 2014; Johannessen *et al.* 2017; Hutchinson *et al.* 2016b). Although families living with YOD are at risk of adverse impacts (Clarke and Hughes 2010), they are often neglected by health and social care service providers (Johannessen and Moller 2013; Barca *et al.* 2014). This failure to provide necessary formal support leads to a range of detrimental effects on immediate and extended family members (Roach *et al.* 2014) across a range of ages and developmental life stages. Effects include impacts on family members' mental health, employment, financial stability and social isolation.

A recent review of service delivery drew attention to policies and practices that frequently fail to address unmet needs and issues of isolation, for individuals living with YOD and their families (Sansoni *et al.* 2016). This has placed higher demands on family members of all ages, at socially significant times in their lives, to provide informal support often at the expense of their own emotional and physical wellbeing (Van Vliet *et al.* 2010a; Roach *et al.* 2014; Hutchinson *et al.* 2016b). The recent Clinical Practice Guidelines for Dementia in Australia pointed out that 'people with younger onset dementia have unique needs and, accordingly, organisations should tailor their services so that they are age appropriate and address the needs of the person with younger onset dementia and their carer(s) and family' (Laver *et al.* 2016: 8).

A gap remains in the literature for the provision of a theoretically informed view on the ways in which societal influences impact the abilities of family members living with YOD to become more visible in society, to live inclusively and equally in their community. So far, broader society does not appear to have an appreciation of the significance of the social environment in the 'disabling experiences of people with dementia' (Keyes 2014: 9; Thomas and Milligan 2018). There is also a lack of appreciation of the fact that socially-constructed disablement is not only experienced by a younger person living with dementia but also by their families. As the needs of younger people with dementia and their families are largely unmet, their experiences of invisibility and disablement can be profound.

## Reflections on the social model of disability as a theoretical lens

The social model of disability has been used extensively in disability research over the years to explain social barriers affecting the rights of those living with impairments and their ability to participate in society. This model draws attention to 'the economic, environmental, and cultural barriers encountered by people who are viewed by others as having some form of impairment – whether physical, sensory or intellectual' (Oliver 2009: 47). It contextualises disablement as a societal responsibility resulting from social exclusion and discrimination (Tregaskis 2002; Oliver 2009; Barnes and Mercer 2011).

Whilst the main focus of the social model has been to tackle disability, through adopting social change and a human rights perspective, there has been much debate amongst researchers as to whether dementia should be linked with disability, similarly to the way in which intellectual and mental health impairments have been (Thomas and Milligan 2018). Even though people with dementia, or others associated with them, do not necessarily identify dementia with disability, they still 'qualify for disability rights and legal protection' (Shakespeare *et al.* 2017; Thomas and Milligan 2018: 118), which would improve their social positioning. However, a 'tendency to over-medicalize' (Shakespeare *et al.* 2017: 4) those living with dementia, focusing on deficits and personal tragedy, has been attributed to the dominance of the biomedical model in service provision. In the biomedical model, living with dementia is defined and described in medical terms, reinforcing disempowerment through an emphasis on how little can be done for people with dementia until there are breakthroughs in medical research. This perspective is challenged by proponents of a social model who consider rights and equality issues for those living with dementia and advocate for inclusive service provision.

In earlier research, we used the social model of disability to explore the lived experiences of children and young people who have a parent with YOD (Hutchinson *et al.* 2016a, 2016b). We found that the children and young people in our study were marginalised, alongside their parent/s, and that they too experienced socially-constructed disablement, a significant factor in the feelings of exclusion and isolation they reported. This persistent disablement resulted in an emotional toll on these young people (Hutchinson *et al.* 2016b). From a social model perspective, to properly support families living with dementia, service providers will be required to shift from an individualistic and isolating view of their lived experiences to a more social context, in which lives are shared and linked with other family members, friends and their community. Taking this viewpoint would improve overall understanding and help tackle the social barriers and discrimination experienced by all those living with YOD, particularly as these relate to different age categories. Adopting this approach would ultimately acknowledge the importance of equal participation and inclusion of the whole family within society (Burchardt 2004; Thomas and Milligan 2015). Taking a social model of disability approach will assist in exploring and understanding experiences of individuals living with YOD, spouse/partners, children/young people and whole families, and better demonstrate the influences of societal barriers and unfavourable attitudes.

The social model is beginning to be used as a research framework for informing service user support in the dementia sector (Gilliard *et al.* 2005; Thomas and

Milligan 2015; Hutchinson *et al.* 2016b). Gilliard and collaborators (2005: 280) described a 'conspiracy of silence', in which healthcare professionals become gate-keepers, unwilling to communicate the diagnosis of dementia and manage the repercussions – just one of the many socially-constructed disablements facing people living with dementia and their families. The Mental Health Foundation in the United Kingdom (2015: 30) recently noted that, although dementia is not viewed routinely as a disability, the social model could be considered useful to 'reframe and reconstruct the world of dementia'. Changing the current way of thinking would not only benefit the rights of the person living with YOD to be supported to live a meaningful life but also support other family members to participate fully in life.

To conceptualise how services can be reframed around the experiences of the service users and their families, we illuminate the complex relationships and experiences of those living with YOD and their families through the lens of the social model of disability, in order to inform service development (Oliver 2009; Gilliard *et al.* 2005).

## The research approach

In this qualitative study, data was obtained through semi-structured interviews with 26 people; five parents under 65 years living with YOD, six partners or spouses of a person living with YOD and 15 children and young people who had a parent living with YOD. Although all the participants in the study belonged to families living with YOD, not all family members participated, and in some families, only one person contributed. Individuals were recruited through Alzheimer's New South Wales, Young Carers New South Wales, the younger onset dementia key worker programme and by the snowball sampling method. The study received ethical approval from the University of Sydney, Australia.

We used the World Health Organization definition of a young person as one between the ages of ten and 24 years. However, the ages of younger family participants ranged from nine to 33 years, and the older of these participants retrospectively described their earlier experiences (up to and including the age of 24). It was anticipated that stories from the past would be recalled and reflected upon from the perspective of their present age and life experiences with a parent living with dementia, and they could then provide insights into how they adjusted to the changes and complex relationships (Hutchinson *et al.* 2016b).

The first author (KH) carried out an introductory phone call or sent an email before conducting the interview and responded to any questions and concerns about the study. KH led face-to-face interviews in the participants' preferred location. Interviews were also conducted by Skype and telephone, so that all interested participants were able to share their stories, regardless of location in Australia. Interviews ranged from one to two hours, with breaks as required, using probing questions. Follow-up phone calls or emails, depending on participants preference, were conducted post interview, and information was provided on organisations and resources that were considered useful.

The three authors familiarised themselves with the data by repeatedly listening to the interviews and reading the interview transcripts to identify recurrent themes and subthemes. The interview data were analysed using a Framework Analysis (Ritchie *et al.* 2013), which is suitable for creating themes from within and between participants (Gale *et al.* 2013). The data was managed using NVivo qualitative data software (NVivo 2012). The research team met regularly to discuss codes and to clarify relationships between codes and group codes. Also develop new codes to account for alternative interpretations of the socio-cultural underpinnings of family and societal experiences, interactions and interventions that shaped family members' experiences of marginalisation and that had contributed to the overarching theme of invisibility. Transcripts were coded into four voice groups: the person with dementia's voice (5), the partner's voice (6), the child/young person voice (15) and child/young person (4) who was the primary carer for their parent. Themes were developed both within and between groups to look at similarities and differences in the family experience. Where possible, transcripts belonging to different members of the same family were also analysed separately and together (4).

This multi-levelled analysis allowed for the development of a better understanding of the whole family experience (Ritchie *et al.* 2007). At this point the theoretical framework of the social model of disability was applied to the dataset and samples were coded by all three members of the research team. Variances with regards to the coding of the data were discussed as a team until an agreement was reached about the thematic coding. The first author then applied this coding to the rest of the dataset. The individuals providing their stories here have been given pseudonyms to retain their anonymity.

## Family experiences of invisibility: interpersonal invisibility

Through the analysis of interview data across different groups of people in families living with YOD, an overarching theme of *invisibility* emerged. This captured their personal experiences of social oppression, isolation and exclusion, all of which shaped interactions within families, with friends and in engaging with broader society. Invisibility appeared grounded in families experiencing socially imposed barriers, including a lack of understanding around living with YOD. Two subthemes also emerged: *interpersonal invisibility*, giving insights into how individual, attitudinal and behavioural barriers impact interactions and relationships between family members, friends and significant others. The second subtheme, *contextual invisibility*, described the way in which specific policies, practices and attitudes adopted by the very organisations and service providers they sought support from, could add to whole family's experiences of isolation, discrimination and marginalisation when living with YOD.

The theme of interpersonal invisibility illustrated social factors that can impact on the relationships of individual family members, parents living with YOD, spouses as caregivers or offspring, as well as in the role of caregivers.

Many participants reported that their needs were not understood, going unrecognised within the whole social context of living with YOD. Their stories highlighted many ways in which they experienced invisibility.

### Sarah, living with YOD

Sarah (42 years old) is married and a mother of four children, aged between nine and 18 years. Sarah described how her diagnosis of YOD, a year ago, had adversely impacted relationships within her family:

> In this house with my husband, flowing down to children, I can say something, and no one listens. It's like I'm not here anymore. I may as well be a cushion or lounge (sofa). Something that needs to be fed, something that talks, my voice has gone.

Sarah shows insights into her enforced dependency in the family, with no opportunity to exhibit choice and control over situations she is part of. This disempowerment has added to her loss of self-esteem and self-worth. She uses the metaphor of herself as a cushion or sofa to describe her feeling that her needs are sat upon, with no one listening to her anymore. These experiences highlight a loss in her personhood as a result of the disabling behaviours and attitudes of significant others in the family. In Sarah's view, her children are modelling her husband's interactions and relationship with her that seems to stem from the medical model, focusing on her deficits and her need to be cared for, rather than the social model targeting her abilities and what she can do.

### Joanne, caregiver

Joanne cares for her husband Fred, diagnosed with YOD at 64 years old. Their two children, one son and one daughter, now in their early 20s, were living at home prior to and at the time of Fred's diagnosis, but at the time of the study had moved out. Joanne reflected personally on how hard the few years were prior to and after Fred's diagnosis. Their son left home due to work and she encouraged her daughter to leave home to 'live the life of a young woman'. Joanne herself was dealing with the changes to her own future, which is often unrecognised.

She ended her career to care for and support Fred, because 'I just want to be with him through this to help him through it because it's just – it's awful'. She describes how difficult this was:

> I was really, really, really struggling because I just felt so alone. So alone and yet so still young and still able to – if we were in a different situation be working full-time and have a really active life … Like how tragic is that?

Joanne lamented the lack of active participation usually associated with her age. Her social isolation and invisibility led to a change in her sense of social connectedness, 'from being a wife to just a carer, and I find that loss of identity really hard to – a real struggle'. Being 'just a carer' gave the sense that this role and change in identity was considered unvalued and insignificant, which contributed to the caregiving role going unrecognised.

From Joanne's perspective, her family was 'amidst the train wreck of our lives'. However, this was not commonly recognised by others in her social circle. For example, a former work colleague asked Joanne, 'how Fred was' but did not ask about her or her family. This confirmed her belief that there was a general lack of understanding that the changed family circumstances with dementia had affected them all. She revealed her difficulty in communicating with others, after experiencing their discomfort and inappropriate responses to her family circumstances; 'how do you tell them what the loss is'? Over time these negative responses caused her to disconnect from family, friends and former work colleagues.

As described by Sarah and Joanne, they felt disconnected and undervalued with the change in their family circumstances. They both highlight problems communicating with their family and friends around their loss, which could contribute to their persistent feeling of being alone. From a medical model perspective, it is the dementia that should be held responsible for their sense of loss and isolation. However, a social model perspective highlights the disabling impact of attitudes and responses to dementia which contributes to their social exclusion and feeling alone.

### Mary and Russell, caregivers

The passage of time can bring new insights, as Russell acknowledged when reflecting on his family experiences with his father, Steven, living with YOD. We spoke to Russell when he was 22 years old, the youngest of four children, and his mother, Mary. Over the previous nine years, since Steven's diagnosis, Russell admitted hiding his feelings, never dealing with his distress associated with his father's deterioration. This contributed to Russell's sense of being alone even though he still lived in the family home. On the other hand, Mary recalls juggling her parenting and caring roles, prioritising everyone else's needs over her own. Mary felt alone and her emotional and physical health deteriorated. Russell, recognising his mother's need for help, remembered how difficult it was to offer support to her while at the same time being overwhelmed himself emotionally: 'I'm dealing with it myself and I can't – I just have to kind of put my arms up and walk away'. Family members, of all ages, living together can find it challenging supporting each other, trying to cope with their own concerns.

This often goes unnoticed by those outside the family, which can ultimately leave people without support options, affecting family connectivity as well as physical and emotional health, as was the case for Russell and Mary. Russell felt he understood Mary's decision to arrange permanent residential care for his father, which Mary acknowledged as a difficult decision. Russell acknowledged the huge demands of caregiving on his mother in addition to other family life pressures, but unknown to his mother, he perceived permanent care as a failure to look after his father, which was hard for him to accept. This had further negative repercussions on Russell's mental health. He described himself as becoming 'really very emotionally unstable. I just got to a point where I was kind of just entirely shutting down kind of emotionally. I was just starting to just seize up and try to just not feel anything anymore'.

An act of self-harm made Russell finally notice his own emotional state, prompting him to acknowledge his need for counselling and support to manage the situation. He admitted he had been hiding his grief from himself, his family and others around him. Russell and Mary's stories demonstrate the importance of maintaining and supporting functional family relationships and connectivity, to keep open avenues of informal support and communication.

### *Beth, sole young carer*

Beth was the primary carer for many years, growing up as the only child to her single mother, Tracey, living with YOD. Beth recalls being eight years of age when there were noticeable changes in her mother's behaviour. They had managed for several years living with her mother's dementia but, when aged 13 years, Beth began 'hanging around with the wrong people' and mentions her 'Mum was too sick to put those boundaries in place'. Extended family members told Beth 'your Mum would be better off if you weren't here. You're just causing more trouble'. Family interventions were unsupportive and harmful at a particularly challenging and vulnerable time of life, triggering Beth to run away from home. This left her isolated from her mother for about a month, which caused, according to Beth, further deterioration in Tracey's mental status: 'I didn't come home because I thought the best thing I can do is to stay away because that's what she (Auntie) told me'.

On Beth's return to live with her mother, the extended family intervened again, taking both Beth and Tracey to live separately with different family members. When she eventually returned to her young carer's role at 14 years, still without either formal or informal support, her mother's condition had progressed. Beth then hid the desperate state of home circumstances for fear of being separated from her mother again, either by the authorities or extended family members. In effect, Beth's fear of asking for help in attempt to safeguard herself and her mother from unwelcome judgements and decisions, contributed to her own and her immediate families' greater social isolation and invisibility.

### *Rachel, sole young carer*

Rachel – the now 27-year-old daughter of a younger person with dementia – reflected on the 16 years looking after her mother with YOD. She felt her situation was invisible to others: 'maybe everyone thought that somebody else was taking care of it or maybe if I was a bit older I would say we need this and I could delegate'.

Rachel felt that her age affected her confidence communicating with adults about what support she and her mother needed. She highlighted a commonly reported situation, in which the views of children and young people were not always taken into account, valued or put into action, resulting in experiences of isolation, hopelessness and vulnerability (Hutchinson *et al.* 2016b). This lack of adequate support and persistent invisibility did eventually take its toll on Rachel. She describes: 'the end of Year 12 when I just started to get worse and worse, really bad depression and self-harming'.

From a social model perspective, the deterioration of Rachel's mental health was not a direct consequence of her mother's cognitive impairment or her young carer role. Rather it appeared to be the general isolation within the family and community, with inadequate formal and informal support, placing barriers to managing the situation well. While participants in this research described a variety of significant relationships with families and their communities, the common thread is one of *invisibility*. These participants illustrate the social barriers that can disable the abilities of families to function well together under complex family circumstances, the social exclusion they face and the general lack of understanding and recognition of their needs to participate fully in life. Rachel and Beth's stories resonated with other young carers' in other circumstances who described themselves as 'the forgotten': young carers say that 'being forgotten, undermined them as people' (McAndrew *et al.* 2012: 16). Consequentially, this demonstrates a disregard for the meeting of their needs and their rights as valued citizens based on their age.

Experiences of social isolation and feeling alone and unvalued negatively impacts all family members in the way they connect, interact and relate to each other and their social world. Our data indicates that consistent support that addresses the needs of individuals and families is necessary to maintain relationships and connectivity within families. Opportunities for meaningful communication for all are crucial in the process of understanding and engaging, ensuring all family members' voices are heard.

## Family experiences of invisibility: contextual invisibility

The theme of *contextual invisibility* highlights factors that impact on interactions and relationships with organisations and healthcare and service providers from whom people seek support and services. This includes the many ways in which people living with YOD and family members feel excluded or unfairly treated based on perceived inequality of services, care and support. In particular, they reported on the tunnel vision of service providers.

### Sarah, YOD

Sarah describes living with YOD as being in a world with a 'tunnel vision' attitude to dementia in younger age. She points out the frequent omission of younger people from dementia-specific research and services, commenting, 'my brain is the same (as older people with dementia), but my age isn't. Really upsets me. Their children have grown up... I feel like a tiny ant waving at people walking around'. By drawing attention to her 'tiny ant' status, Sarah demonstrates her sense of unimportance, as well as her insignificance and the discrimination against her within the world of dementia research and dementia sector. Barriers based on age and diagnosis should not be an inevitable part of living with YOD and need readdressing. The social model perspective supports the non-discriminatory right to be treated equally and be given the same rights and opportunities as others.

### Phoebe, YOD

Phoebe, diagnosed with Lewy body dementia at 49, has been living alone with formal supports since her diagnosis. She described how her diagnosis was negatively portrayed by a health professional:

> Everyone has a choice when you're given a diagnosis. When I was given my diagnosis, it was basically an end of life diagnosis like, okay, you need power of attorney. Get – do an advanced medical directive and go home and wait to die.

Based on the medical response to her diagnosis, Phoebe felt worthless and disempowered, deprived of the freedom of choice on her right to life. She defined her diagnosis of YOD as the 'invisible disease', feeling this explained behaviours of fear and avoidance attributed to the lack of understanding, which led to experiences of stigma and marginalisation. Fortunately, a positive experience with both a geriatrician and a psychologist 'undid the end of life diagnosis and said you can do anything you want to do'. This brought about a positive change in her overall attitude, promoting freedom and autonomy to live life as she chose, and she then went on to become an advocate for others living with YOD. Phoebe's healthcare providers initially focused on her deficits: her life was over and she should prepare for end-of-life care. From a social model perspective, the attitudes of clinicians should help portray her situation more optimistically, supporting her right to be actively involved in decision-making, to engage in life and focus on the things she was capable of and not on her deficits. Examples like these serve to illustrate the disabling nature of the medical model, which often fails to recognise people living with YOD as having the human right to choose, take part in supported decision-making and actively participate in society.

### Joanne, caregiver

Joanne had personal experience of caring for a family member with cancer, as well as her husband, Fred, living with YOD. She discussed the disparity between carer education and services offered by the dementia sector, compared with the cancer sector. Joanne's observations reflected those of other participants, in emphasising the invisibility of their situation where service provision appeared to be siloed around diagnostic labels, rather than need. Joanne summarised these feelings:

> because of the education around cancer, everyone gets it, they understand it, there's no stigma around it, there's incredible support. Cancer has such a high profile, and people get it, but with Alzheimer's it's – yeah, they think it's something that's lurking there that's waiting to pounce on you.

### *Freya, caregiver*

Freya is one of two children providing care for her single mother, Grace, living with YOD. She used the words 'hidden disease' when talking about her mother's life with YOD in comparison with the experiences with her father, James, who had terminal cancer. Freya noted disparities in the way people communicated, often ignoring her mother, but engaging with her father, asking after his health. These opposing responses could stem from the more significant public awareness or public profile attached to cancer over dementia, and the ambiguity surrounding YOD, which fails to see people living with YOD as active citizens with rights.

Joanne and Freya, from different families but both caregivers, have experienced first-hand the negative impact of a label of dementia, influenced by a lack of community education and awareness and understanding around the experience of YOD. It is important that dementia sectors globally disseminate information more widely, to make YOD more visible. Inclusive education is required to help change attitudes and improve responses and service opportunities, particularly for those of a younger age. The successful approaches implemented by the cancer sector to increase profile and visibility could potentially be adopted and modified by the dementia sector.

## Navigating support and service as sole carer for a parent

Navigating a complex system with little support and direction adds to the overall distress of families living through the progression of cognitive impairment. Participants of all ages revealed their traumatic experiences when deciding to place the person with YOD into permanent residential care, as is consistent with other studies (Bakker *et al.* 2010; Barca *et al.* 2014; Cabote *et al.* 2015). Once the decision is made, the process to identify a suitable facility for someone under 65 years is challenging and often leads to further anguish on the part of family members.

### Rachel, young carer

When Rachel was in her early 20s, she was faced with the daunting task of obtaining permanent residential care for her mother in a location near where she lived. She recalled her frustration:

> I just don't know where people want me to go. I go to dementia specific, they don't want me there. Well, that's what Mum's got so then I go another place, and they won't have me there. I can't travel to Wollongong to go to the younger persons place, and I don't think I'll be able to get her in. So I want her close to me, and I don't know what to do.

Rachel cried with overwhelming relief when her mother was finally accepted into a good quality permanent residential care home. For many years Rachel's life had revolved around caring for her mother with little external support, but the opportunity of living autonomously was now a possibility for Rachel, who phrased this as 'this is my world and Mum's world is separate'. Rachel was finally able to be a daughter again, rather than a full-time carer, and adopt a healthier lifestyle, to 'do sport, I exercise every day, and I can plan my meals out. It's just so much better'. The lack of understanding of family circumstances and needs on the part of agencies charged with assisting people such as Rachel, had left her unsupported and battling a complex system to obtain the necessary formal care for her mother. In this way, Rachel had been experiencing socially-constructed disablement that limited her ability to participate in daily activities that many people take for granted, such as exercise and social interaction with peers.

## Young carers' support can be a 'lifesaver'

Suitable services and supports can be challenging to find or access, and service availability varies with location. With the added complexity that most services do not adopt a family approach, young carers are often not visible to service providers. This contributes to most children and young people believing they are alone in their experiences of having a parent with YOD, which adds to their sense of difference and isolation. For some, having opportunities for sharing personal experiences and meeting with other young people facing similar life situations, is helpful. Rachel joined a group where she could meet other young people with parents living with dementia and referred to this group as a 'lifesaver': 'I think the best thing that's happened was meeting those young people that are in the same boat because I think the problem with Alzheimer's is that nobody understands'.

Young people described the benefits of being noticed and afforded proper attention, specific to individual need and age. With this recognition, they felt empowered and more able to cope with changing family circumstances. Also, being considered as belonging to the family by people providing formal services improved their overall self-worth and value, which others have also reported (McAndrew *et al.* 2012).

Social isolation and exclusion is a shared experience with family members living with YOD. It is a consequence of the failure to recognise the rights of everyone in the family to have equal access to services and supports, relevant to their age and situation. Reframing of dementia as a social concern would influence the way in which services were designed and how families engage and respond to services and support being modelled around need, not a diagnosis. Also, adopting this social approach could be the impetus for change in policy and practice within health and social care, to help remove social barriers, enabling choice and control, offering alternative approaches and responses (MHF 2015).

## Implications of 'invisibility' in families living with younger onset dementia

Our findings illustrate how the complexity of interactions and relationships within families living with YOD, their social circle and with their service providers, can impact in such a way that they experience disablement, irrespective of the extent of their impairment. The ability to engage in experiences similar to other families or even in a way that is socially consistent with the stage in their lives, can be considerably impeded by their social oppression, isolation and exclusion. The theme of *interpersonal invisibility* highlights the complexity of maintaining meaningful relationships and connections with family members and significant others when lives deviate from their expected trajectory. Often, individual needs remain unrecognised and unmet based on negative attitudes and a lack of understanding of YOD, thus adding to their disablement. *Contextual invisibility* exposes the impacts of organisations, particularly health and social care providers, in the experiences of exclusion, disablement and isolation of family members. Current policies and practices can contribute to denying the rights for full participation and inclusion in society, based on the persistence of the medical model approach to dementia.

The experiences presented in this study demonstrate that feelings of isolation, marginalisation and exclusion by all family members, are socially constructed. The cognitive impairment from YOD in these cases did not explicitly, nor directly, lead to invisibility, but rather the reactions of individuals across the range of social contexts within which these families lived. Consequently, each family member's capacity to function and adapt to ongoing complicated circumstances in their lives was dependent on their ability to maintain healthy and supportive relationships, within the family and with significant others. The capacity of a family to support each other's needs and function well together can be dependent on receiving family-centred formal support, services and information that recognises needs across ages.

## Reflections on ways forward

One approach through which to overcome the invisibility of family members and their capacity to support each other, be supported and to function together, relates to understanding previous family functioning (La Fontaine and Oyebode 2014; Roach *et al.* 2014). There can be internal negotiation within families around caregiving and support, but the success of this can be contingent. Its outcomes are not predictable: it may create greater intimacy within the family or exacerbate distance (Carpentier *et al.* 2010: 1502). Our findings indicate that the experience of isolation for family members living with YOD stems from marginalisation, discrimination and a general lack of understanding: their experiences often go unacknowledged by both formal caregivers and other family members. This can deter young people from sourcing information that might be helpful (McAndrew *et al.* 2012; McDonald *et al.* 2016). Meeting the needs of families to both access and be able to share information could sustain positive informal family support and reduce the risk of emotional distress (Svanberg *et al.* 2010; Roach *et al.* 2014; McDonald *et al.* 2016).

Interviews with family members demonstrated the relationship between lack of social support or negative social support and psychological wellbeing, leading to the mental distress reported by Brodaty and Donkin (2009). Specialised practical and emotional support for the whole family, that acknowledges the influence of family history and connected lives, is necessary throughout the progression of the dementia. This will undoubtedly help to reduce overall strain, improve capabilities of all family members to cope with a changing life course and improve future outlook (Carpentier *et al.* 2010; Johannessen *et al.* 2017).

To be effective, services and resources available need to be designed and delivered in ways that are responsive to, and mindful of, changing needs, circumstances and challenges faced by each specific family. A sense of inclusion and being valued within one's family remains essential, arguably more so when one member is living with dementia. This can promote each family member's emotional wellbeing and sense of self (Harris and Keady 2009; Hutchinson *et al.* 2016b). This is particularly relevant for the person with YOD, who becomes more vulnerable over time, and thus feels increasingly disempowered and without a voice. A sense of inclusion is also especially important for children and young people in these families, who can feel insignificant and excluded because of their age (Smyth *et al.* 2011; McAndrew *et al.* 2012; Barca *et al.* 2014).

Despite this tendency to overlook children and young people, they are at times still expected to navigate complex systems and advocate for services on behalf of their parent with YOD, without any acknowledgement by healthcare and social care providers of their existence within the family (Hutchinson *et al.* 2016a). Their experiences and viewpoints can also be disregarded and dismissed by older family members, even when they are the primary caregiver for their parent. Family members, friends, healthcare and social care providers need to be more aware and mindful of the vital role children and young people play in keeping the family together and functioning, and in providing mutual support. Greater understanding of their roles will help in the inclusion of their needs in family focused service design and development (McAndrew *et al.* 2012; Hutchinson *et al.* 2016a, 2016b).

Family breakdown and conflict are real concerns; fragmented families lose informal support options, leaving individual family members more isolated. The combination of limited in-family support and inadequate formal support options can, in some cases, hasten the admission of the person with YOD to residential care. This is one of the most stressful and emotionally distressing transitions for families living with dementia (Allen *et al.* 2009; Lockeridge and Simpson 2012). Poor management of invisibility and complex family circumstances can, for some family members, instigate the development or worsen already present mental health issues. A family-focused approach is essential to recognising and responding to the age-based needs of all family members so that they receive adequate, timely and ongoing formal support and guidance (Millenaar *et al.* 2016; Sansoni *et al.* 2016; Cations *et al.* 2017). Only in this way can needs be recognised and family crises averted.

Avoidance and discriminatory behaviours by other family members, significant others and service providers, causes people to feel invisible, adding to their distress. Family members can lose their sense of self and togetherness: life spins out of control without proper attention from family, friends and formal support networks (Roach *et al.* 2014; Hutchinson *et al.* 2016b). Changing roles and responsibilities, such as becoming a caregiver within the family, affects self-identity and emotional wellbeing, especially if these changes have been imposed without choice and control, and are not acknowledged by others. Family members then experience 'fear, loss and abandonment' (Harris and Keady 2009: 442), affecting their ability to cope and adjust to difficult and unexpected challenges: a diagnosis of YOD comes at a point in life when this circumstance is rarely anticipated. The resulting social disablement, as in Russell's case above, may trigger a decline in one's mental health, creating further difficulties (Tew *et al.* 2012). This deterioration in mental health can also be considered as socially-constructed disablement, directly related to the stresses experienced as a result of the inadequate social support and lack of supportive connections within the family and with significant others (Lockeridge and Simpson 2012).

## Changing service provision and enabling families

Improving the visibility of people living with YOD and their family members is a social concern. We have drawn attention to the socially-constructed disablement that results from their invisibility that acts as a barrier to participating as equals in society. Awareness of these disabling factors will direct the change needed to design and develop family-focused services that affirm the non-discriminatory rights of all members of these families.

The under-representation of people and families living with YOD continues to be evident in research. This is a major contributing factor in the experiences of invisibility for those living with YOD. As a consequence, the development of dedicated services are rare for these families (Brown *et al.* 2012: 8; Millenaar *et al.* 2016), because of the lack of awareness of their specific needs. Lack of appropriate support enhances isolation, marginalisation and inequality.

We argue that this lack of support can be addressed in a large part by adopting the social model of disability. Dementia has not been considered a good fit with this model but recent studies are highlighting its relevance across the whole trajectory of dementia (MHF 2015; Thomas and Milligan 2018). The social model promotes choice, decision-making and control over the way one participates in life. Many people living with dementia are now recognising this as their right and are advocating for more equality (MHF 2015). The social model of disability clearly identifies the failure to identify and provide for families living with YOD, addressing age-appropriate services and support, as a barrier to social equity and inclusion.

Considering there is currently a dearth of services, a paradigm shift is necessary. This requires moving away from the present focus on deficits and what people living with dementia cannot do – the focus of the medical model – to embracing a can-do approach and the right of choice in everyday life, under a social model. Reframing services and support to be socially-orientated would mean people living with YOD and their families would be recognised and supported based on their needs, and actively involved in the process of change. No longer would their circumstances be considered a personal tragedy, where nothing can be done and they become passive recipients of services. Negative attitudes towards impairments are barriers to social equality and inclusion, as the social model of disability identifies (Thomas and Milligan 2015). Bringing about attitudinal change is crucial and will be facilitated through creating opportunities for all people affected by a diagnosis 'to communicate and interact' (Wenger 2000: 232). These opportunities will deepen the societal understanding of experiences living with YOD. Supporting positive interactions can be the foundation for making the invisible features of living with YOD visible, thereby bringing attention to how society currently disables these families from participating fully in life.

To make the invisible visible, there needs to be leadership to drive the change, committed to renegotiating opportunities, connecting people to share experiences, including communicating needs and offering tangible and tailored support (Wenger 2000). This could be accomplished through the backing of the dementia sector, but needs cross-sector cooperation to take in awareness of the range of ages of family members involved. Implementing a fully-inclusive approach would enable families living with YOD to participate in public and health awareness strategies without judgement and discrimination.

It is well known that discriminatory attitudes to impairments are disabling, as highlighted in disability research. This needs to be addressed in policy, even if challenging (Fisher and Purcal 2017). Social attitudes towards those with dementia can result in oppressive and exclusionary practices (Thomas and Milligan 2018), often based on misunderstandings, general lack of knowledge and the undervaluing of difference. However, the dementia sector and dementia-related policies have been slow in adopting a social approach to dementia because of the dominance of the biomedical model (MHF 2015). We must learn from and adopt practices to raise awareness of dementia as has been done in the disability and mental health sectors, so as to improve the right to inclusion and equality for the whole family (Beresford *et al.* 2010; Barnes and Mercer 2011; Oliver 2013). We know that the practice of diminishing social barriers requires a multifaceted approach (Fisher and Purcal 2017).

The inclusion of the families living with YOD will be essential to effective public raising awareness campaigns advocating for more social contact with families living with YOD in the community, to improve familiarity with dementia and for education programmes across schools and various organisations including health and in the community. Children, the future citizens, can be informed about dementia through specifically-designed education programmes at schools, which will assist in changing perceptions of dementia and promote a dementia-inclusive society (Baker *et al.* 2017).

It is crucial that attention is drawn to the whole family's needs, regardless of age, so that people are no longer disabled by their invisibility. The parent with YOD is an integral family member, so the entire family should be enabled to function together and be fully supported to participate in life. Roach and collaborators (2014: 1414) have argued that 'the way the family functions can ultimately impact the life of the person with dementia and how the person living with dementia experiences their diagnosis can impact how the family functions'. This supports the view that all family members should be identified at the outset of any service provision and their input into informing specific family-focused services and support must become routine (La Fontaine and Oyebode 2014). Adopting a cross-sectorial collaborative approach with family members would ensure that no one is left alone, isolated and uninformed; ultimately assisting them to remain connected to the family and be routinely informed of support options to improve experiences of living with YOD.

Changes in approaches to service provision could be facilitated through development and implementation of ongoing education and training programmes with a social model focus. Healthcare professionals participating in education programmes, which provide valuable real-life insights into the many social factors that create barriers to families living with YOD, would hopefully embrace a social approach to dementia in their practice. This would help in the process of removing these barriers. Shifting the focus from deficits of YOD, as described by Phoebe, can bring hope that life is worth living and can enable the family to actively engage in life with dementia, with the necessary support. For some healthcare and social care providers, this will involve becoming more aware of their own need to explore and overcome their negative perceptions of dementia (Edwards *et al.* 2014). This greater self-awareness may help them adopt a more enabling approach in their practice, improve interactions with families and provide greater job satisfaction.

## In conclusion

Dementia research, policies and practices need to unify dementia within the broader context of societal relations and responsibilities rather than simply treating it as a diagnosis. This should include more innovative strategies for raising awareness of the experiences of dementia in younger people and their family members. Age is a significant factor in living with YOD, a major contributor to explaining the invisibility of all family members. Taking a social model approach to YOD will shift societal perceptions; better inform policy and practice changes; optimise service development and interactions; and promote enablement and inclusion of all family members living with YOD.

Dementia sectors are becoming more responsive and inclusive of all types of dementia. They now need to address the perceived insignificance of those with YOD and their family members, so that no one feels like 'a tiny ant'. Collaborative development and implementation of health and community education and activities to raise awareness will assist challenge the negating and unfavourable views of dementia and thus eliminate social barriers. Collectively these advancements will be an impetus to countering family experiences of socially-constructed disablement when living with YOD, promoting greater visibility in the community. Reframing YOD will ultimately improve the health and wellbeing of all family members, acknowledge their rights to services and supports based on need and irrespective of age, in turn enabling their feelings of social inclusion.

## References

Allen, J., J. Oyebode, J. Allen, 2009, Having a father with young onset dementia: The impact on the well being of young people, *Dementia*, 8: 455–480.

Baker, J., J. Yun-Hee, B. Goodenough, L. Lee-Fay, C. Bryden, K. Hutchinson, L. Richards, 2017, What do children need to know about dementia?: The perspectives of children and people with personal experience of dementia, *International Psychogeriatrics*, 1–12.

Bakker, C., M. De Vugt, M. Vernooij-Dassen, D. Van Vliet, F. Verhey, R. Koopmans, 2010, Needs in early onset dementia: A qualitative case from the NeedYD study, *American Journal of Alzheimer's Disease and Other Dementias*, 25(8): 634–640.

Barca, M., K. Thorsen, K. Engedal, P. Haugan, A. Johannessen, 2014, Nobody asked me how I felt: Experiences of adult children of persons with younger onset dementia, *International Psychogeriatrics*, 26(12): 1935–1944.

Barnes, C., G. Mercer, 2011, *Exploring Disability*, Cambridge, UK: Polity Press.

Beresford, P., M. Nettle, R. Perring, 2010, Towards a social model of madness and distress? Exploring what service users say, *Joseph Rowntree Foundation*, www.jrf.org.uk/report/towards-social-model-madness-and-distress-exploring-what-service-users-say.

Brodaty, H., M. Donkin, 2009, Family caregivers of people with dementia, *Dialogues in Clinical Science*, 11: 217–228.

Brown, J., K. Sait, A. Meltzer, K. Fisher, D. Thompson, R. Faine, 2012, *Service and Support Requirements of People with Younger Onset Dementia and their Families*, Sydney, Australia: Alzheimer's Australia.

Burchardt, T., 2004, Capabilities and disability: The capabilities framework and the social model of disability, *Disability and Society*, 19: 735–751.

Cabote, C., M. Bramble, D. McCann, 2015, Family caregivers' experiences of caring for a relative with younger onset dementia: A qualitative systematic review. *Journal of Family Nursing*, 1-26.

Carpentier, N., P. Bernard, A. Grenier, N. Guberman, 2010, Using the life course perspective to study the entry into the illness trajectory: The perspective of caregivers of people with Alzheimer's disease, *Social Science and Medicine*, 70: 1501–1508.

Cations, M., A. Withall, R. Horsfall, N. Denham, F. White, J. Trollor, B. Draper, 2017, Why aren't people with young onset dementia and their supporters using formal services?: Results from the INSPIRED study, *PLoS ONE*, 12(7): 1–15.

Clarke, H., N. Hughes, 2010, Introduction: Family minded policy and whole family practice – Developing a critical research framework, *Social Policy and Society*, 9: 527–531.

Edwards, R., S. Voss, S. Iliffe, 2014, Education about dementia in primary care: Is person- centredness the key? *Dementia*, 13: 111–119.

Fisher, K., C. Purcal, 2017, Policies to change attitudes to people with disabilities, *Scandinavian Journal of Disability Research*, 19(2): 161–174.

Gale, N., G. Heath, E. Cameron, S. Rashid, S. Redwood, 2013, Using the framework method for analysis of qualitative data in multi-disciplinary research, *BMC Medical Research Methodology*, 13: 117.

Gelman, C., C. Greer, 2011, Young children in early onset alzheimer's disease families: Research gaps and emerging services needs, *American Journal of Alzheimers Disease and Other Dementias*, 26: 29–35.

Gilliard, J., R. Means, A. Beattie, G. Daker-White, 2005, Dementia care in England and the social model of disability: Lessons and issues, *Dementia*, 4: 571–586.

Hall, M., P. Sikes, 2016, From 'what the hell is going on?' to the 'mushy middle ground' to 'getting used to a new normal': Young people's biographical narratives around navigating parental dementia, *Illness, Crisis and Loss*, 0(0): 1–21.

Harris, P., J. Keady, 2009, Selfhood in younger onset dementia: Transitions and testimonies, *Aging and Mental Health*, 13: 437–444.

Hutchinson, K., C. Roberts, M. Daly, C. Bulsara, S. Kurrle, 2016a, Empowerment of young people who have a parent living with dementia: A social model perspective, *International Psychogeriatrics*, 28: 657–668.

Hutchinson, K., C. Roberts, S. Kurrle, M. Daly, 2016b, The emotional wellbeing of young people having a parent with younger onset dementia, *Dementia*, 15: 609–628.

Johannessen, A., A. Moller, 2013, Experiences of persons with early onset dementia in everyday life: A qualitative study, *Dementia*, 12: 410–424.

Johannessen, A., K. Engedal, K. Thorsen, 2016, Coping efforts and resilience among adult children who grew up with a parent with young-onset dementia: A qualitative follow-up study, *International Journal of Qualitative Studies on Health and Wellbeing,* 11(1): 30535

Johannessen, A., A. Helvik, K. Engedal, K. Thorsen, 2017, Experiences and needs of spouses of persons with young-onset frontotemporal lobe dementia during the progression of the disease, *Scandinavian Journal of Caring Science*, 31(4): 779–788.

Keyes, S., 2014, Ageing, in K. Wharton (ed.), *Disability Studies*, First edition, London: Sage Publications.

La Fontaine, J., J. Oyebode, 2014, Family relationships and dementia: A synthesis of qualitative research including the person with dementia, *Ageing and Society*, 34: 1243–1272.

Lambert, M., H. Bickel, M. Prince, L. Fratiglioni, E. Von Strauss, D. Frydecka, E. Reynish, 2014, Estimating the burden of early onset dementia: Systematic review of disease prevalence, *European Journal of Neurology*, 21(4): 1–7.

Laver, K., R.G. Cumming, S.M. Dyer, M.R. Agar, K.J. Anstey, E. Beattie, H. Brodaty, T. Broe, L. Clemson, M. Crotty, M. Dietz, B.M. Draper, L. Flicker, M. Friel, L.M. Heuzenroeder, S. Koch, S. Kurrle, R. Nay, C.D. Pond, J. Thompson, Y. Santalucia, C. Whitehead, M.W. Yates, 2016, Clinical Practice Guidelines for Dementia in Australia, *Medical Journal of Australia*, 204: 191–193.

Lockeridge, S., J. Simpson, 2012, The experience of caring for a partner with younger onset dementia: How younger carers cope, *Dementia*, 12: 635–651.

Mayrhofer, A., E. Mathie, J. Mckeown, F. Bunn, C. Goodman, 2017, Age-appropriate services for people diagnosed with young onset dementia (YOD): A systematic review, *Aging and Mental Health*, 1–9.

McAndrew, S., T. Warne, D. Fallon, P. Moran, 2012, Young, gifted and caring: A project narrative of young carers, their mental health, and getting them involved in education, research and practice, *International Journal of Mental Health Nursing*, 21: 12–19.

McDonald, F., P. Patterson, K. White, P. Butow, I. Costad, I. Kerridge, 2016, Correlates of unmet needs and psychological distress in adolescents and young adults who have a parent diagnosed with cancer, *Psycho-Oncology*, 25: 447–454.

Mental Health Foundation (MHF), 2015, Dementia, rights, and the social model of disability, Policy discussion paper, *Joseph Rowntree Foundation*, www.mentalhealth.org.uk/publications/dementia-rights-and-social-model-disability.

Millenaar, J., C. Bakker, R. Koopmans, F. Verhey, A. Kurz, M. De Vugt, 2016, The care needs and experiences with the use of services of people with young-onset dementia and their caregivers: A systematic review, *International Journal of Geriatric Psychiatry*, 31(12): 1261–1276.

NVivo, 2012, *NVivo Qualitative Data Analysis Software (Version 10)*, London: QSR International Pty Ltd.

Oliver, M., 2009, *Understanding disability from theory to practise*, Basingstoke, UK: Palgrave Macmillan.

Oliver, M., 2013, The social model of disability: Thirty years on, *Disability and Society*, 28(7): 1024–1026.

Ritchie, J., L. Spencer, W. O'Connor, 2007, Carrying out qualitative analysis, in J. Ritchie and J. Lewis (eds), *Qualitative Research Practice: A guide for social science students and researchers*, London: Sage.

Ritchie, J., J. Lewis, C. Nicholls, R. Ormston, 2013, *Qualitative Research Practice: A Guide for Social Science Students and Researchers*, London: Sage.

Roach, P., J. Keady, P. Bee, S. Williams, 2014, 'We can't keep going on like this': Identifying family storylines in young onset dementia, *Ageing and Society*, 34: 1397–1426.

Sansoni, J., C. Duncan, P. Grootemaat, J. Capell, P. Samsa, A. Westera, 2016, Younger onset dementia: A review of the lierature to inform service development, *American Journal of Alzheimer's Disease and Other Dementias*, 31(8): 693–705.

Shakespeare, T., H. Zeilig, P. Mittler, 2017, Rights in mind: Thinking differently about dementia and disability, *Dementia*. (Epub ahead of print)

Smyth, C., M. Blaxland, B. Cass, 2011, 'So that's how I found out I was a young carer and that I actually had been a carer most of my life': Identifying and supporting hidden young carers, *Journal of Youth Studies*, 14: 145–160.

Spreadbury, J., C. Kipps, 2017, Measuring younger onset dementia: What the literature reveals about 'lived experiences' for patients and caregivers, *Dementia*, 1–20.

Svanberg, E., A. Spector, J. Stott, 2010, 'Just helping': Children living with a parent with young onset dementia, *Aging and Mental Health*, 14: 740–751.

Svanberg, E., A. Spector, J. Stott, 2011, The impact of young onset dementia on the family: A literature review, *International Psychogeriatrics*, 23: 358–371.

Tew, J., S. Ramon, M. Slade, V. Bird, J. Melton, C. Le Boutillier, 2012, Social factors and recovery from mental health difficulties: A review of the evidence, *British Journal of Social Work*, 42: 443–460.

Thomas, C., C. Milligan, 2015, How can and should UK society adjust to dementia? (ref: 3132), *Joseph Rowntree Foundation*, www.jrf.org.uk/report/how-can-and-should-uk-society-adjust-dementia.

Thomas, C., C. Milligan, 2018, Dementia, disability rights and disablism: Understanding the social position of people living with dementia, *Disability and Society*, 33(1): 115–131.

Tregaskis, C., 2002, Social Model Theory: The story so far, *Disability and Society*, 17: 457–470.

Van Vliet, D., C. Bakker, R. Koopmans, M. Vernooij-Dassen, F. Verhey, M. de Vugt, 2010a, Research protocol of the NeedYD-study (Needs in Young onset Dementia): A prospective cohort study on the needs and course of early onset dementia, *BMC geriatrics*, 10: 13–13.

Van Vliet, D., M. De Vugt, C. Bakker, R. Koopmans, F. Verhey, 2010b, Impact of early onset dementia on caregivers: A review. *International Journal of Geriatric Psychiatry*, 25, 1091-1100.

Wenger, E., 2000, Communities of practise and social learning systems, *Organisation*, 7: 225–246.

# 5 Generational perceptions of dementia in the public sphere

## Public health, age-othering and generational intelligence

*Simon Biggs, Irja Haapala and Ashley Carr*

## Introduction

Dementia is increasingly being discussed in the public domain as population ageing increases the number of people living with dementia, making it a health, social and economic policy issue (Prince *et al.* 2015). These public discussions often exist against a background of negative attitudes towards ageing and media-generated rivalry between generations. Simultaneously, in public discourse, dementia is seen as an extreme version of the worst aspects of ageing and the most feared endpoint to the life-course (Ballenger 2006: 107; Léon *et al.* 2015), and the relationship between ageing and dementia has become blurred (Scodellaro and Pin 2013; Cahill *et al.* 2015). In shaping this public discussion, age-based attitudes towards dementia are an important focus for changing wider public opinion. However, there is a gap in current research evidence, in that it does not allow for an examination of age-based views of dementia. A consideration of age difference as it effects the reception of public health messaging, might provoke a rethink of how campaigns are targeted. Particularly if it increasingly takes into account the position of the recipient.

In this chapter, we examine age group differences in perceptions of dementia, the relationship between attitudes towards ageing and towards dementia, drawing on our research and existing research literature in the fields of social gerontology and public health. Conceptually, this relies on an examination of age-othering, the process of seeing the other person as someone who is constructed as being of a different group to oneself, within the particular context of ageing and dementia and intergenerational relationships and the possibility of increasing understanding between age groups.

Throughout this chapter, we use dementia as an umbrella term to refer to all different types of progressive neurological conditions affecting the brain (Winblad *et al.* 2016). While dementias consist of a number of diverse conditions, in the public mind these frequently exist as a common and simplified condition, under the word 'dementia', as reflected in a variety of public health surveys. Further, people tend to collapse 'age' and 'dementia', thus provoking an embedded and inflated sense of otherness and denial of the condition, especially among those affected at a younger age. This places the examination of public perceptions of dementia within the context of wider social ageism, making intergenerational understanding a doubly difficult, but not insurmountable, challenge.

We argue, in the context of social ageing, that public perceptions of dementia are an extreme form of othering associated with age. We introduce a theoretical framework of generational intelligence (Biggs and Lowenstein 2011; Biggs *et al.* 2011) as a means to address the connection between age and dementia in the public domain. Then we focus on recent reports from public surveys on the association between age and public knowledge of and attitudes towards dementia, presenting results from our research on age-based differences in perception. To conclude, we bring the discussion back to the issue of othering, looking into ways in which we might increase intergenerational understandings in future public health campaigning.

## Ageing and 'othering'

The notion of 'othering' has been used in a number of discourses on difference, including gender and ethnicity, to describe the process by which social antagonisms become manifest in interpersonal perception and behaviour (Bernasconi 2012). People's attitudes towards ageing, at a personal and social level can, according to Biggs *et al.*, result in a particular form of othering between social actors. An 'Age-Other' is,

> someone who is constructed as being of a different group to oneself, based on age. Age-otherness may include aspects of life-course, family position and cohort identity. Whether an individual is seen as being 'other' will be affected by the interaction of these elements of generational identity.
>
> (2011: 1108)

Age-based othering has most commonly been thought of as a negative phenomenon:

> Every individual has the potential to experience discrimination or prejudice based on their age if they live long enough. It produces an 'othering' effect that lumps all those considered old into a category defined, first, as different and, secondly as inferior. More importantly, it suggests that all old people are alike, hence obscuring differences that exist among and between older persons.
>
> (Phillips *et al.* 2010: 21)

We are dealing with a complex set of socially-created cognitive and emotional associations with ageing, interacting differently with one another as we ourselves age. This constitutes what Bollas (1989) argues is a transition from simple to complex thinking that begins in mid-life; in younger years, all are perceived either as of the same or strikingly different age from one's own. With negative othering, the vacuum created by an absence of intergenerational connection is filled by negative, social stereotypes simply because they, instead of the positive ones, are readily available in wider society. Ageism is a longstanding phenomenon (Marshall 2007; Moody 2008) that, among other social issues, has been associated with intergenerational rivalry (Kohli 2005) and as an excuse to reduce benefits to older adults (Minkler and Robertson 1991; Williamson *et al.* 2003; Grattan Institute 2014; Intergenerational Foundation 2015). The understanding of dementia as a social issue, therefore, sits within a series of debates and public discussion about ageing and generational relations that may reinforce negative othering and reduce progress to forms of empathic understanding.

## 'Othering' in relation to dementia in public discourse

In public discourse, dementia constitutes an extreme form of othering associated with ageing. This is manifest in a number of negative representations in the public sphere. Negative othering in relation to dementia can easily be reinforced and perpetuated by language used by the most vocal or visible people: politicians, celebrities and others in positions of power or who we look up to (Gerritsen *et al.* 2016). Perhaps among the most potent representation is an association between the supposed behaviour of zombies in popular culture and the social space created for dementia (Behuniak 2011). In emotional-psychological terms both are connected with horror: disgust at decay and a fear of being devoured. Behuniak calls this a 'dehumanisation based on disgust and terror' leading to 'a politics of revulsion and fear' (2011: 70). Zelig (2014) takes this further, connecting anxiety about old age and mental illness with the politics of individualism and social disintegration, which we simultaneously have to live with and distance ourselves from.

We argue that such representations or descriptions should not be seen as a metaphor, explaining dementia to the uninitiated, but rather as a contribution to the creation of a narrative space in which the two images – zombies and people living with dementia – become merged. Unfortunately, in public discourse, this narrative can easily take hold and the two images become almost indistinguishable in their psychological and social meaning, and their stigma can be feared for contamination by close association. To counter such narratives, the importance of the public sphere as a place to influence public perception on ageing and dementia and to break down barriers to intergenerational empathy has become ever stronger since the broad uptake and use of social media and media overall (Van Gorp *et al.* 2012).

Strengthening of intergenerational empathy in the public sphere will serve as a positive link between public perceptions of ageing and dementia and a bridge to positive othering associated with dementia. We see this as a bridge in so far as most of us will grow old, and therefore the likelihood for each of us of becoming the other is significantly enhanced. In the case of othering related to dementia, however, the question would be how far a state that appears to be so radically 'not me' now, can leverage the prospect of 'me in the future' when the present narrative represents a person one has no desire to be. Intergenerational acknowledgement of dementia as a public health and personal risk, across generations, may be the first step towards empathic understanding in this case.

## Generational intelligence and empathic understanding

One way the question of the connection between othering and age difference has been addressed is through the framework of generational intelligence, described by Biggs and Lowenstein (2011) and Biggs *et al.* (2011), as a means of interpreting the degree of empathy arising between generational groups. Encountering an 'age-other' is seen as comprising three dimensions: the degree to which one becomes conscious of self as part of a distinctive age group, the relative ability to put oneself in the position of other generations and a relative ability to negotiate between generational positions. The salience of each element will vary depending on context, and the views of each age group are shaped by a combination of social forces and personal experiences which, under the right circumstances, are capable of critical revision by the viewer. A high level of generational intelligence reflects an ability to take multiple perspectives into account and engage in meaningful communication between age-groups, while a low level reflects a reduced willingness or ability to put oneself in the position of the age-other (Haapala *et al.* 2015). This approach has been used by Dow and collaborators (2016) with Melbournian elders and young people and with Hong Kong nursing students to successfully enhance positive age perspective-taking in dementia care (Au *et al.* in press). We use this framework to discuss age-based views on dementia as reported by public health surveys and our qualitative research.

Taken together, our view is that a critical analysis of public discourse on ageing and dementia should include an examination of attitudes and views among generationally-distinctive age groups. This is particularly important in the case where people living with dementia are doubly 'othered' – once through the lens of ageing and then through the lens of the condition itself.

## Public health challenge

Public attitudes towards dementia have become important as dementia has become a global public health priority (World Health Organization 2012, 2016). Dementia has risen to this status partly because of the sheer number of people affected by the condition as populations across the globe age, but also because dementia can be considered on par with cardiovascular disease, diabetes and cancer, as a public health issue, in so far as they can increasingly be prevented, staved off or stalled by individual action on the modifiable risk factors, i.e. changes in lifestyle (Winblad *et al.* 2016; Kivipelto *et al.* 2017; Livingston *et al.* 2017). However, this public health message is rarely acted on, most likely due to lack of research evidence on the effectiveness of lifestyle interventions and people's capabilities to adhere to the suggested changes in lifestyle. For people to change their lifestyle, as explained by most health promotion theories, they must first become aware of their personal risk and the behaviours at stake, but also trust in their own capabilities to change and believe that the suggested change is effective and advantageous for them personally (Brownson *et al.* 2015). To date, public health campaigns in relation to dementia have focused on raising awareness of the condition at the population level. Their effectiveness, or reception, can best be assessed via large-scale surveys on public knowledge and perceptions. For us, this gives an opportunity to continue our exploration into age-based othering of dementia, by examining the current research on public views on and attitudes toward dementia, particularly among different adult age groups.

We have found that most of the research concentrates on survey data, reporting on the extent to which the general population (18 years and above) are aware of dementia, that it is a chronic disease rather than a natural part of ageing, and their overall knowledge about the condition. Findings indicate that dementia remains largely unknown, something to do with older people and ageing, and that little can be done about it or one's personal risk (Cahill *et al.* 2015; Livingston *et al.* 2017; Prince 2017).

Only a few studies have focused on age differences when reporting on knowledge and attitudes towards dementia; even then, results are often aggregated over too wide an age range to allow for age group comparisons. Phillipson and colleagues (2014) reported that among 616 respondents between 40 and 65 years in Australia, age was associated with valuing the person with dementia (reported as person-centredness), but no other information on age-related attitudes was reported. Likewise, Cheston *et al.* (2016) collected data from 794 individuals representing four adult age-groups (16–24 years, 25–49 years, 50–64 years, 65 years and over) in England, yet only respondents above and below 65 years were identified in the reported results that showed 'younger people' (64 years and less) to hold more positive attitudes (hope and recognition of personhood) towards dementia than 'older people' (65 years and above) did. While both of the above studies report the positive effect of personal contact and providing help, support or care for someone with dementia, data has not been analysed by age or age group in this regard. In terms of age group differences in attitudes, overall the findings of these two studies are contradictory. This, in our mind, leaves scope for a closer analysis of the effect of age, but may indicate some positive attitudes towards dementia across all adult age groups.

When age group differences are reported, either the research approach or method adopted may not allow for further in-depth analysis of the responses. This applies to an Irish study reported by Glynn *et al.* (2017), which indicated that in a sample of 1217 survey respondents, those in the younger age group (15–39 years) were consistently less likely to answer correctly statements assessing general knowledge on dementia, its risk factors, prevention options and its link with ageing, when compared with the other age groups (40–59 years and 60 years and above). Close to half of the younger age group believed that dementia was a normal part of getting older or affected only those above 65 years, whereas this view was shared by only one-third of the respondents aged 60 years and older. These findings suggest that the younger age groups in Ireland could use more information on dementia and that their perception of personal risk and the link between ageing and dementia may lead to negative othering of dementia, but again, the research method does not allow for closer analysis of age group differences in this regard.

Similar results have been reported by Alzheimer Europe (2011) from a survey conducted in four European countries plus the United States ($n$=499–639), showing that fear of dementia was highest among those aged 60 and over (20 per cent to 47 per cent of respondents in the five countries), and lowest among 18–34-year-old respondents (6 per cent to 22 per cent). Léon *et al.* (2015), in an assessment of the effect of the French National Dementia Plan 2008–2013 ($n$=2013+$n$=2509), reported that, in 2013, 71 per cent of respondents aged 65 years and older reported fear and were the most concerned about dementia (seriousness, fear, lack of information or feeling embarrassment in the presence of people with dementia, 39 per cent to 71 per cent across variables) when compared with those aged 18–34 years or 35–64 years (fear reported by 44 per cent and 57.6 per cent, respectively). While this study showed that those who had provided care for a person with dementia (13.8 per cent) felt more informed and less embarrassed in the interaction, the age of the respondent was not taken into account. In the French sample, dementia was considered by 69.1 per cent of all respondents in 2013 to be a normal part of ageing, a common misconception held by the public. In addition, these studies suggest that among age groups below 60–65 years, a perception of low personal risk of dementia is prevalent, which allows people to move the condition further away from self (as in othering) and that the level of understanding of dementia as a chronic condition may be insufficient even among those aged 65 years and over.

Smith and colleagues' (2014) survey of 20–75 years old Australians ($n$=1003) found people over 60 years showing more knowledge and concern about dementia than the two younger age groups (23–39 years and 40–59 years), but less likely to believe that risk reduction should start before the age of 40 years (44.4 per cent versus 65.7 per cent and 56.3 per cent, respectively). Only 2.2 per cent (23–39 years) and 5 per cent (40–59 years) rated dementia as an important health issue for them to have information about, whereas for 17.2 per cent of people over 60 years it was one of the two most important health issues. The younger age groups ranked cardiovascular disease, stress and obesity as the three most important, which is useful information for public health campaign/intervention designers in relation to dementia, due to their role as modifiable risk factors for dementia (Livingston *et al.* 2017). In this Australian sample, only 41.5 per cent strongly believed that their risk of dementia could be reduced, which indicates a need for more understanding of the condition and its risk factors. In terms of our search for age group specific views on dementia and age-based othering of dementia, this study implied more understanding among the younger adults, although direct comparison cannot be done due to different questions and research aims. While the study provides valuable data on age group specific attitudes, it is based upon survey data, and focuses more on risk prevention than attitudes towards ageing and dementia.

This brief overview of age-specific public knowledge and perceptions of dementia indicates that research has rarely taken a life-course (longitudinal) or generational (age groups) approach that would show in the reporting of results. Age appears mainly as a distinction between those above or below 60 to 65 years, with findings based on answers to pre-defined survey questions aimed at discovering receptiveness of existing public health campaigns and priorities. A more nuanced approach to age-based perceptions by age groups might enhance the understanding of past public health campaigns and interventions and lend support to future ones, especially if research suggests that specific age-groups perceive dementia differently and thus may be receptive to particular messaging priorities. We suggest that the degree to which one can put oneself in the place of the age-other, when that distinction is perceived to be radically different from one's own, could be key to the effectiveness of future public interventions on issues aimed at influencing attitudes related to dementia. We engage with this question next, examining findings from our qualitative research into public perceptions of dementia, with a particular focus on differences in views by the adult age-group, and examine how these might reflect 'othering', generational understanding and empathic understanding.

# The research[1]

## *Methods and participants*

Here we report findings from qualitative in-depth interviews of 29 self-selected people from healthcare (*n*=4), social work (*n*=5) and service professions (including hairdressers, IT and media consultants, hospitality and customer service staff) (*n*=20), recruited via aged and dementia care-related professional and consumer organisations and with invitation cards placed in community-centres, local cafes and shops. Participants were interviewed in 2017 as part of our research into public perceptions of dementia. To answer the conceptual questions of age difference in perceptions, othering and generational understanding, we have analysed the data by age group.

Table 5.1 presents a summary of participants' gender, age, professional field and contact with dementia (knowing or providing informal care for someone with dementia within or outside the family) by age group. In this sample, the younger adults' age group had contact with dementia only through work, whereas 60 per cent to 62.5 per cent of participants in each of the other age groups had this contact within the family and many provided care/support, but were not the primary care/support person (Table 5.1). Most of our participants (75.9 per cent) were born in Australia and seven (24.1 per cent) overseas. Participants born overseas had lived in Australia for an average of $29.4 \pm 21.9$ years (between 7.5–59 years) and only three spoke a language other than English at home. Our sample is not representative of the Australian population: the 2011 Australian Census reported 26 per cent born overseas, and 19 per cent aged five years and over spoke a language other than English at home.

During semi-structured telephone interviews, lasting for approximately one hour, with open-ended questions, we probed the interviewees to speak about

Table 5.1 Participant characteristics by age group

| Characteristics | Age group (years) and number of participants | | | | |
|---|---|---|---|---|---|
| | Younger adults (18–35 y) (n = 6) | Mid-life (36–50 y) (n = 8) | Later mid-life (51–65 y) (n = 10) | Older adults (66+ y) (n = 5) | Total (n = 29) |
| Gender | | | | | |
| Men (n) | 0 | 2 | 3 | 1 | 6 |
| Women (n) | 6 | 6 | 7 | 4 | 23 |
| Age (years) | | | | | |
| Mean | 30.8 | 46.3 | 56.8 | 69.0 | 50.6 |
| Min–max | 25–35 | 40–50 | 51–64 | 67–71 | 25–71 |
| Professional field | | | | | |
| Healthcare professions | 3 | 1 | | | 4 |
| Social work professions | 2 | | 1 | 2 | 5 |
| Service professions | 1 | 7 | 9 | 3 | 20 |
| Contact with dementia | | | | | |
| Yes, helps with care within family | | 2 | 2 | 2 | 6 |
| Yes, knows someone within family | | 3 | 4 | 1 | 8 |
| Yes, outside the family/through work | 6 | 2 | 4 | 2 | 14 |
| No, does not personally know anyone with dementia | | 1 | | | 1 |

their personal views on five main themes: first thoughts about dementia as a condition, public perceptions and generational difference, main challenges, personal priorities and campaigns related to the condition. In this chapter, we report on responses to four of the probing questions, under two themes.

First thoughts on dementia. Here we asked two questions: when I say 'dementia', what do you think about?; and to what degree is it a normal part of ageing? These were designed to provide us with the participant's immediate response to the 'other' and to elicit views on ageing and its association with dementia.

Public perception and generational difference. Here we report on two questions: how do you think dementia is perceived by people in the street?; and how do you think the perceptions might differ between generational groups? These posed the question of age difference as a factor in critical reflection. For a more detailed methodological description, see in Haapala *et al.* (in press).

Transcripts were independently coded by two researchers with a high level of inter-coder reliability and nine themes emerging from the first thoughts on dementia were further categorised according to the tone of the response, carrying either a negative, positive or neutral tone, e.g. describing the condition purely as biomedical or physiological symptoms, plus age-related views which were often neutral in tone: empathy (positive tone), cognitive loss (neutral tone), elderly/older people, younger people also affected (age-related), sadness/loss, loss of the person, fear at personal level, overall negative issues and terminal nature of the condition (negative tone) (Table 5.2, p. 76). Validity of the coding process was supported by researcher triangulation between the two coder-interviewers and the principal investigator plus consultation with the advisory group of the dementia research consumer network. Participants' views on whether dementia was a normal part of ageing were coded as Yes, No and Partly yes/Not sure (Table 5.3, p. 77). Themes emerging from the coded responses to the second and third question (public perceptions and generational difference) were examined using narrative analysis and cross-tabulated with first thoughts to examine difference within and between age groups (Table 5.4, pp. 84–85). After exporting descriptive query matrices from NVivo, to identify major emphases within each age group, further narrative analysis of each question followed our conceptual framework to identify age-othering and generational understanding/empathic understanding by age group.

## Findings

Responses to the four questions are summarised below and interpreted according to the age-group of the participants, and conceptual issues including age-othering and empathic understanding.

### *First thoughts on dementia*

Table 5.2 presents a summary of the first thoughts expressed by our interviewees in each age group. The tone of the response (neutral, age-related, negative or positive) is also indicated. In response to our first question, most interviewees in

Table 5.2 First thoughts expressed, by theme and tone of response. Number and percentage (%) of first thoughts expressed, categorised into nine themes with a negative, positive or neutral tone of the response indicated by age group

| Themes | Age group | | | | |
|---|---|---|---|---|---|
| | Younger adults (18–35 y) (n = 6) | Mid-life (36–50 y) (n = 8) | Later mid-life (51–65 y) (n = 10) | Older adults (66 y +) (n = 5) | Total (n = 29) |
| Positive tone: empathy | 2 (15.4) | 2 (15.4) | 2 (11.1) | 1 (16.7) | 6 (14.0) |
| Neutral tone: cognitive loss | 5 (38.5) | 6 (46.2) | 7 (38.9) | 3 (50.0) | 21 (42.0) |
| Age-related: elderly/older people | 1 (7.7) | 1 (7.7) | 2 (11.1) | 0 | 4 (8.0) |
| Age-related: younger people | 1 (7.7) | 0 | 1 (5.6) | 0 | 2 (4.0) |
| Negative tone: sadness/loss | 1 (7.7) | 2 (15.4) | 2 (11.1) | 1 (16.7) | 6 (12.0) |
| Loss of the person | 2 (15.4) | 0 | 2 (11.1) | 0 | 4 (8.0) |
| Fear, personal | 1 (7.7) | 0 | 1 (5.6) | 1 (16.7) | 3 (6.0) |
| Negative, overall | 0 | 2 (15.4) | 0 | 0 | 2 (4.0) |
| Progressive to death | 0 | 0 | 1 (5.6) | 0 | 1 (2.0) |
| Total number of first thoughts, n (%) | 13 (100) | 13 (100) | 18 (100) | 6 (100) | 50 (100) |

each of the four age groups spoke about dementia in neutral terms, reflecting different types of the condition, changes in brain activity and other physiological or biomedical issues (38.5 per cent to 50 per cent of the first thoughts within age group).

First thoughts with a negative tone constituted roughly one-third of the views in each of the four age groups (30.8 per cent to 33.3 per cent). The three younger age groups reflected on the impact on the person and others, particularly families and expressed sadness related to the condition, while in the older adults' age group, negative thoughts centred on overall sadness and fear at a personal level. The mid-life age group also mentioned difficulties with care and support services. Positive comments, i.e. empathy for the people affected by the condition, were expressed by all age groups, surpassed by age-related thoughts only in the later mid-life age group. Age-related thoughts, either related to older adults or also younger people, were mentioned (by 7.7 per cent to 16.7 per cent of the interviewees) in the three younger age groups, but not at all in the older age group. This was also reflected in the way our interviewees responded to the question about the link between dementia and ageing: older adults and younger adults were mostly of the opinion that dementia is not part of normal ageing, while this was not the case in the two middle age groups (Table 5.3).

Taken together, where the age groups differed, was the extent to which their views expressed empathy and concern plus age-related thoughts, reflecting the interviewee's distance to the condition. Distance, lacking contact or experience with the condition or distancing oneself from the condition, was related to age of the viewer and the extent and type of contact with dementia they had experienced. Closer narrative analysis of the first thoughts revealed subtle differences according to age, as detailed below.

Younger Adults (*n*=6) in our sample, had experienced contact with people with dementia only through their professional work. This may explain why their first thoughts reflected a mixture of age-related distance or professional role-related distance, tempered by elements of emotional empathy.

*Table 5.3* Can dementia be considered a normal part of ageing? Responses are coded into three categories, Yes, No, Not sure/partly yes, according to age group

| | | Age group | | | | Total |
|---|---|---|---|---|---|---|
| | | *Younger adults (18–35 y)* | *Early mid-life (36–50 y)* | *Later mid-life (51–65 y)* | *Older adults (66+ y)* | |
| Yes | *n* (%) | 1 (16.7) | 2 (25.0) | 4 (40.0) | 1 (20.0) | 8 (27.6) |
| No | *n* (%) | 4 (66.7) | 4 (50.0) | 5 (50.0) | 3 (60.0) | 16 (55.2) |
| Not sure/partly yes | *n* (%) | 1 (16.7) | 2 (25.0) | 1 (10.0) | 1 (20.0) | 5 (17.2) |
| Total | *n* (%) | 6 (100.0) | 8 (100.0) | 10 (100.0) | 5 (100.0) | 29 (100.0) |

A sense of distance from the condition was expressed by Zoe (25 years old), who stated: 'I've never come across it before, so it's quite foreign to me. A great unknown', referring to real-life situations as opposed to dementia training. Likewise, Ruby's (35 years old) views reflected distance to the condition when she referred to the impact of dementia on families, saying that 'I couldn't imagine being in that situation. Hard for the families to lose the person they've known previously'. Thinking of younger onset dementia, Nancy (35 years old) saw dementia as 'Really tragic for people with young onset dementia. Just really sad, because they become different people, they are not themselves'.

Young adults' personal contact with dementia (through family/friends) may have enabled a particular kind of empathy to emerge. Most of the first thoughts in this age group expressed sympathy for the family of a person with dementia. For Zoe (25 years old), empathy emerged through reflection on her own situation: 'you kind of think that [this] could happen to my family or that could happen to me … and fear of not knowing what to do or not knowing how to deal with someone like that'. Getting to know individuals with dementia through a dance class, Anita (33 years old) expressed an understanding of the cognitive challenges, which could differ from individual to individual:

> I think about someone who's lost their full cognitive functions but is still perhaps able to have the concepts in their mind, they're just not able to spit them out … some people can formulate things well and they just perhaps can't remember a certain section, whereas, others it's a little bit more difficult.

While younger adults responded to the emotional effects of dementia on themselves and others, this had rarely been experienced in relationships. Rather it was something that affected others: people with dementia and those around them, but the condition was not seen as something that affected only older adults and neither was it linked with ageing. Only one in six (16.7 per cent) interviewees in this age group saw dementia as a normal part of ageing, linking it with genetics and lifestyle choice:

> I would say it's a pretty normal part of ageing, I just think some people get more, yeah, predisposed to dementia than others and for some people probably their brains will always function up until the end, like, they're not predisposed to that or they're not predisposed to having any sort of issues with their brain function and they've probably looked after themselves. And that impacted on them being able to live life without any big issues coming up, like dementia.
>
> (Chloe, 33 years old)

For the other five in this age group, the following quote from Jessica (28 years old) is illustrative:

I don't think it is the normal aging process. I think the more common it becomes, the more people are inclined to think of it as normal aging. But I certainly am of the opinion that it's not. It's a pathological process that's abnormal and it doesn't happen to everyone.

In the Mid-life group (*n*=8), views were divided about dementia being a normal part of ageing or not and many (25 per cent) were uncertain, unlike in the younger adults' age group where the predominant view was that dementia is a disease/pathological process. When, in the mid-life age group, dementia was considered even partly as normal part of ageing, a thought like this one by Sally (47 years old), is illustrative: 'It is a normal part of ageing. A body system thing that – I don't know – I guess the brain wears out'. In this age group, the thoughts on normal/disease process did not vary by contact with dementia (data not included here).

Not unlike the younger adults, mid-lifers viewed dementia as from a distance, as something not affecting their age group at the personal level. However, their first thoughts were more neutral, focusing on cognitive, descriptive thoughts about physiological changes and the negative impacts of the condition. As Sally (47 years old), knowing someone with dementia in the family, suggested:

I think about not being able to carry out normal daily actions and functions, not being able to function normally in the world ... being impeded in actually doing things in the world. When I think of dementia I think of regression, I think of immobility, hospitalisation, and often poor care homes.

Emma (47 years old), currently providing care for a family member with dementia, but also working outside of home, gave a descriptive account, of 'knowing that someone has gone from a normal life to slowly progressing, not knowing family members, not being to tie shoelaces, just daily basic functions they can't do'.

Dementia was, as Cameron (50 years old), pointed out when reflecting on his family history, something that affected older adults: 'So with my nana ... what we witnessed was someone who could not do a lot for themselves, who ... could not really understand things and could get frustrated easily'.

Mid-lifers' neutral and cognitive first thoughts enabled them to comment on the current state of care homes, lack of resources and cost of care. Brendon (47 years old) thought about those that have 'to take care of those people with dementia', and the expense 'for society because of the [level of] support required'. Amber (43 years old) reflected on 'hospitalisation and care' and 'being put away' in nursing homes. Mid-lifers, then, tended to think in terms of othering the issue, moving it away from self, to affect society, carers and people affected by dementia rather than it affecting themselves. Their reactions were descriptive and reflected a sense of the other in which emotions rarely find expression.

In the Later Mid-life group (*n*=10), an increasing amount of contact with dementia was evident, and their first thoughts, while being mostly neutral, focused also on negative impacts and were personal and communicative in orientation. Those without or with limited experience of people with dementia expressed first thoughts that reflected a sense of distance, based on their own lack of knowledge rather than their age or life-course position. And, for later mid-lifers without experience of dementia within the family, when interaction did occur, the reactions varied from easy-going to more emotional. Ivan (52 years old) responded in a practical and thoughtful way: 'on the few occasions I've had to deal with people you fairly quickly become quite patient and be prepared to go around in circles at times, but that's okay', while Francesca (61 years old), when confronted by residents with dementia in 'nursing homes ... carrying dolls or things like that', thought of the situation as 'sad and a bit hard'.

Participants in this age group were most likely of all age groups to consider dementia to be a normal part of ageing: 40 per cent (16.7 per cent to 25 per cent in the other age groups) reflected a 'yes' response. However, often dementia was considered as forgetfulness, as illustrated by Rosemary (56 years old), currently providing care for a family member with dementia, but also working outside of home: 'Yes. As they get older, I think, life becomes slower, their mind becomes slower, urgency isn't there and I think forgetting things is just part of that'.

Nevertheless, when it was not considered normal by interviewees in this age group, it was still associated with increasing age as the biggest risk factor, as Scott (61 years old) said: 'No. Chances go up, but no'.

In this age group, interviewees were also more likely to reflect on their personal ageing and the likelihood of themselves developing dementia. This was particularly the case for those with contact with dementia within the family. As Frank (55 years old), currently providing care for a family member with dementia, but also working outside of home, stated:

> I'd say it's frightening ... I think at my age, I feel, hey, am I going to take after my father? Is that me in 25 years' time? So, there is that, there's a fear there, I think that's of the whole thing, and, you know, and, if you forget something, you think you're getting dementia, you know.

In the later mid-life group, the pronouns 'they' and 'them', used by younger age groups, were often replaced with 'you' and 'I', indicating more closeness to the age at which dementia was seen to be unavoidable part of life. Mavis (64 years old), for example, commented: 'I think, now I'd say the decline of *your* memory, and eventually you say irreversible and terminal illness; *you* will lose *your* power to eat and lose *your* power to speak'.

Those with a care connection also drew on experience of a significant other as their main reference point. 'I think with dementia ... and I'm probably talking more about my father ... You can't reason with someone with dementia because there's not that understanding anymore' (Rosemary, 56 years old).

While these responses saw dementia as 'other', a narrative of association through personal ageing and the importance of communicative ability appeared, which was uncommon among younger age-groups.

The Older Adults age group ($n=5$), increasingly drew on the day-to-day challenges of dementia, and the implications for relationships as compared with other age-groups. Lloyd (69 years old) described dementia as 'less ability to do the normal, daily things of movement and getting around'. In a similar way, Sylvia (67 years old) commented first-hand about the daily challenges, describing dementia as 'difficulty with everyday tasks' followed by reflecting on the experience of 'a challenging, frustrating, often debilitating, unknown journey'. Dementia is framed as a personal, but unpredictable journey, rather than a 'great unknown'. Both Lloyd and Sylvia represent here the voice of professionals without family contact with dementia.

Among interviewees in this age group, for those who had contact with dementia through the family, in particular, the condition held immediacy as part of one's personal ageing: 'It frightens me that I might end up with it', stated Brenda (68 years old), in what was typical of this age group. However, they were on par with the younger adults (60 per cent and 66.7 per cent, respectively) to see dementia as a pathological condition and disease rather than a normal part of ageing. Only some considered it normal, as Heidi (71 years old) put it: 'to some degree it's a normal part of aging but I don't think people understand that as well'.

The older adults' group were the only ones to remark directly on the need for empathy. Angela (70 years old), currently participating in the care of a family member with dementia, commented:

> The first thing I'd think about is empathy, the need for help. It's really hard, because knowing the things I know, the first things I think about is how can I make this person happy, and that's one of the things that is my daily goal, is to make people happy.

Angela also raised the issue of inclusion, the need for social contact and the experience of being shunned: 'once they have that diagnosis and people know about it, they tend to move away, drop off and not want to communicate'. In this context, Heidi (71 years old) described an individual with dementia as 'somebody who is losing their memory capacity and their quality of life', reflecting on her thoughts that:

> anybody with dementia should be doing and given the opportunity to do as they want to. It might not mean that they've got to spend money; it might only mean that they actually go gardening; just be happy and enjoy it.

For most of the interviewees in the older adults' age group, the person with dementia was a real person rather than an 'other'; dementia was less distant, more personalised and tied to direct experience, more so than for the interviewees in other age groups.

## Views on public perception and generational difference

All age groups in our sample saw the public perception of dementia as negative and believed that knowledge of the condition was low. However, there were minor differences in emphasis, typical of each age group.

Younger Adults (*n*=6) were more likely to suggest that dementia was viewed by the general public as a mental health issue that was hidden from public view. As Chloe (33 years old) stated: 'I suppose people can go, "Well, they've probably got mental health" and move on. I think it's a very hidden problem and you can't see the disability front-on'.

Mid-lifers (*n*=8) commented on a general lack of understanding, with implications for how people in public interact and relate to people with dementia. As Bonnie (48 years old) implied, unease among the general public with talking about dementia could result in people thinking that little could be done about dementia:

> They don't understand it, so they just don't talk about it, or they are very uneasy talking about it. They don't know a lot about it, they just see it as it's portrayed in the media, as a terrible disease that causes death.

This suggests that people tended to respond not to real situations but in the 'same old stereotyped manner', as Cameron (50 years old) added.

Later Mid-lifers' (*n*=10) views on public perceptions reflected greater diversity than evident in other age groups. Some suggested the persistence of fear, as stated by Alice (51 years old): 'I think people are horrified by it. Well, they're scared of it'. Others commented on people's desire to avoid the topic, as Mavis (64 years old) said: 'Most of my friends they don't like, when I hit the topic and then they want to change the topic'. Despite these negative views some believed that greater understanding was emerging and evident: 'I think most people are fairly compassionate and understanding about it' (Ivan, 52 years old).

Older Adults (*n*=5) were distinctive in focusing on the stigma associated with dementia and the negative reactions that could result. Heidi (71 years old) thought that dementia 'still has a stigma involved', which she 'wanted to see broken down so that it [dementia] comes out in the open'. Sylvia (67 years old) identified stereotypes and avoidance, and said that people saw dementia 'As an embarrassment'. Others pointed out the prevailing negative and inaccurate views on dementia, which led to fear:

> They're as scared as hell of it. They sort of shy away from it. Because a lot of information that comes out [in the media] about dementia is about the behaviours, people think, oh, they're going to get aggravated, and they're going to hit me, and they're going to do this, and you know, people don't understand the condition.
>
> (Angela, 70 years old)

Each age group identified personal contact as an antidote to dementia stereotypes in the public sphere. Three examples are typical: Anita (33 years old) suggested that 'unless they know someone who's been affected they really don't know much about it'; Erin (48 years old) believed that 'Dementia would not even cross their mind unless they had some personal connection'; and Francesca (61 years old) said, 'Unless they have had experience with it, like a grandparent or whatever, I think they would find it – how would you word it – sort of – they'd find those people a bit weird'.

To summarise the findings presented above, we have prepared Table 5.4 which includes the age group specific *first thoughts, views on public perception* and what will be described next as the *generational differences in perceptions* of what our interviewees thought their own age group and other age groups currently think about dementia. What becomes interesting is how each age group perceives their own age group's perceptions when compared with their own first thoughts on dementia.

## Perceptions of younger adults' views

When we asked our interviewees to consider how specific generational groups responded to dementia in the public sphere, the responses from all of the four age groups were in agreement that younger adults paid little attention to dementia and that awareness increased with age. Younger adults felt that their own age group would not have much interest in dementia unless there was some real-life contact through family or work: 'They are so far removed', stated Zoe (25 years old), and 'don't really think anything bad is going to happen to [them]' with only 'direct family experience' acting to counter this situation. Young adults in our sample were employed in helping professions, which may set them apart from what they themselves consider an 'average young adult'. Both mid-life age groups and older adults shared this view of the younger adult group, and added that even though they might be better educated, younger adults could be dismissive, seeing dementia as a concern for older adults only, and as a source of humour or ridicule. Nevertheless, personal experience through family or friends was assumed to increase positive perceptions even though the general view was assumed to be negative and ageist.

## Perceptions of both mid-life age groups' views

Little distinction was made by our interviewees between the perceptions held by mid-lifers and later mid-lifers. Only the later mid-life age group saw mid-lifers, as opposed to their own age group, as in greater denial of their personal risk and as less ready to talk about the condition; a view which later mid-lifers attributed also to older adults. While young adults saw no difference between mid-lifers' and their own age group's views, they assumed awareness and interest in dementia to be dependent on personal (family) contact: 'Mid-lifers would have no interest without real-life or personal contact' (Ruby, 31 years old), the other

Table 5.4 First thoughts and views on public perceptions of dementia by age group

| | Younger adults (n = 6) | Mid-life (n = 8) | Later mid-life (n = 10) | Older adults (n = 5) |
|---|---|---|---|---|
| First thoughts | Neutral with empathy; distant, recognising risk starting earlier in life<br><br>Not linked with ageing | Neutral; sadness and empathy, thinking of negative impacts, some distance<br><br>Can be a normal part of ageing | Neutral; sadness and empathy, concerned about negative impacts at personal level; less distant<br><br>Can be a normal part of ageing | Neutral; empathy, sadness and fear; less distant<br><br>Not a normal part of ageing |
| *Views on public perceptions of dementia among:* | | | | |
| The general public | Negative; sad, mental health issue, forgetfulness, or short-term memory loss | Negative; madness in old age; lack of understanding and skills to interact, perhaps understanding is on the rise | Negative; ageist, feared, level of knowledge and understanding is dependent on personal contact among family or friends, denial or avoidance, some compassion, but less stigmatising than before | Negative; mental health issues or on drugs, intoxicated, ageism and stigma attached, feared because of media portrayal, embarrassment within families, scared/shy away from it, not acknowledged, invisible, lack of understanding and awareness |
| Younger adults | Personal contact dependent, otherwise, not much interest | Personal contact dependent, otherwise, not much interest | Personal contact dependent, otherwise, not much interest; may be more educated about it; dismissive and consider it a low personal risk, associate it with age | Personal contact dependent, otherwise, not much interest; dismissive of personal/familial risk; might laugh at it, misunderstand as depression or part of ageing |

| | | | | |
|---|---|---|---|---|
| Mid-lifers | 'Same as us' | Personal contact dependent, but overall more aware; many have contact through family or friends' family; wondering about own memory and behaviour; interested in health but too busy to engage | Personal contact dependent; fear but seek information only as needed, busy elsewhere; denial of personal risk ('not me'); not ready to talk about it; 'Same as older adults' | Personal contact dependent, otherwise, not much interest; easily dismissive or in denial; starting to notice and consider need for personal lifestyle changes; resourceful in helping people living with dementia |
| Adults in later mid-life | 'Same as mid-lifers and us' | 'Same as us' | Personal contact dependent; link it with ageing, often see it as unavoidable part of ageing; trying to avoid and prevent it | 'Same as mid-lifers' |
| Older adults | Potentially a lot more real for older adults | Great concern due to higher prevalence; more interest in health issues; fear due to inadequate knowledge level and media portrayal | 'Same as mid-lifers (but not like us)' | Personal contact dependent, otherwise, no thought given to it; main target group; find it hard to manage if affected; concerned and alarmed; if believe in 'no cure', then remain in denial |

three age groups saw mid-lifers as being generally more aware of dementia (than younger adults), possibly due to having parents or friends' parents experiencing the condition. However, they were thought to be too busy with other issues to pay it much attention. As expressed by one of the interviewees in the mid-life age group, Bonnie (48 years old), the mid-life cohort today was 'a little bit more open to new ideas and ways of thinking', but that they were 'not as supportive as older ones, because they just don't have the time'.

Mid-lifers added to this view of their own age group by suggesting that mid-lifers were concerned with their own mental and physical health, overall. Similarly, later mid-lifers added that their own age group, as opposed to younger mid-lifers, were most likely to be engaged in informal care and that many would see dementia as an unavoidable part of ageing and either try and avoid it or hope to prevent it in some way. For example, Ivan (52 years old) stated that later mid-lifers are 'probably a bit more sympathetic to their [people living with dementia] situation because you see it as potentially something you'll have to deal with', referring to provision of care. Alice (51 years old) further added that, 'I think a lot of middle-aged people are caring for their elderly parents, and so they're probably faced with it and they probably just find it sad and scary', and Francesca (61 years old) thought that 'as you get older, I think, because you're getting closer towards that possibility, or personally might be at risk, there is a bit more understanding or caring about those things'.

In terms of denial, Mavis (64 years old) suggested that: 'young adults and mid-lifers, they think, it will never happen to me', and Heidi (71 years old) felt that both mid-lifers and older adults were driven by avoidance: 'mid-lifers [both early and late mid-life] and older adults think, because I can't deal with it so I don't want to know'. Nevertheless, several older adults saw mid-lifers as resourceful in their support for people living with dementia: 'People in middle age have got the expertise ... I think that generation can be more resourceful in their support for people, rather than older generations' (Sylvia, 67 years old).

Again, personal experience of dementia through family or friends emerged as a factor enhancing positive perceptions, but within an overall tendency towards avoidance or concern over personal risk.

## Perceptions of older adults' views

Other age groups perceived that older adults' age-based proximity made dementia 'potentially more real' (Zoe, 25 years old) and easier to cope with, as they were seen as 'far more tolerant, accommodating and aware of it' (Nancy, 35 years old) and as having 'more insight because they generally have peers who are starting to experience it' (Megan, 40 years old). In contrast, older adults themselves saw their age-peers as often either in denial or increasingly concerned and struggling to cope if faced with the condition. Yet they saw their own age group as most at risk. Sylvia (67 years old) pointed out that this age group, because of lack of knowledge, 'usually think it's a form of depression or anxiety, or mental health, and say, she'll recover from it, get over it'. Brenda (68 years old) saw this age group as 'quite concerned and alarmed' and Angela (70 years old) said they were 'secretly concerned', adding that 'it's, in particular, when you have someone in the family that's been diagnosed with dementia', referring to older couples trying to cope with it on their own.

The overall view of this age group was that they were assumed to be more familiar with dementia. They also were thought to have a heightened level of concern accompanied by not knowing how to cope. Personal contact with dementia through family or friends again emerged as an assumed mediator to a more positive perception and there was a mismatch between what older people themselves thought and this public view.

In summary, and in reference to Table 5.4, when the interviewees' first thoughts and the above attributions to age-based views in the public sphere are compared, it is striking how different an age-group's own views on dementia contrast with what they think their peers among the general public might think. Their own views are more nuanced and less stereotyped. This, together with a common expectation that personal contact rebuffs social stereotypes, offers some hope that generational perceptions of dementia are mutable and open to change, reducing age-otherness and increasing empathic understanding.

## Discussion and conclusions

This chapter has focused on a conceptual analysis of othering, the process of seeing the other person as someone who is constructed as being of a different group to oneself, within the particular context of ageing and dementia. We have examined this in relation to age group differences in perceptions of dementia, with the possibility of increasing empathy and understanding of dementia across age groups. Three salient findings are detailed below with further suggestions for age-based analysis of understanding of dementia, othering and empathy between generational groups.

First, this data confirms that age-differences can be expected in the perception and responsiveness to dementia as a socially-constructed category. As suggested by a generational intelligence approach, empathy varied by age group. While younger adults showed a form of distanced empathy, mid-lifers saw the other from a predominantly cognitive viewpoint, and later mid-lifers as an other encountered in practical communication. Older adults exhibited a set of attitudes closer to the self and based on interaction with others. Often these responses evidenced benign forms of othering, that it was not really connected to them.

All age groups described current public perceptions as negative. These differences indicate the importance of a shift in emphasis for public health intervention from assessing the reception of pre-defined messaging, to an awareness of where recipients are in terms of age-based priorities and life-course position. While more extensive study is called for, age should be considered an important element in the perception of dementia and how messages are responded to. Indeed, the persistence of age differences across topics in the current study argues for a more finely tuned targeting of interventions, by adult age or generation.

Second, while there were elements of distancing, there was minimal evidence of negative othering within our sample. People with dementia were othered in, for example, the use of the pronoun 'they', the lack of narrative connection between self and other and in that dementia was not seen as a positive life-course development. However, understanding of dementia was often sympathetic, especially where there was or had been some form of personal or family connection with dementia in the past. Further, the focus of understanding varied between the four age groups we studied, with younger adults showing greater emotional empathy, yet lack of significant contact; mid-lifers focusing on cognitive understanding and service issues; later mid-lifers on communication; and older adults on forms of interpersonal connection. These foci were not mutually exclusive but did, we would argue, reflect differences in life-course priorities and experience.

Third, empathy appears to have become enhanced by forms of personal connection and contact with dementia through family or friends. Interest in dementia may not otherwise appear on one's personal radar. Generational empathy, as in our sample, may be reflected in sadness and concern for families among younger adults, displaced onto knowledge and prevention amongst mid-lifers and reflected in concern for communication and interaction amongst the two older groups. Our findings are in agreement with Phillipson *et al.* (2014), Léon *et al.* (2015) and Cheston *et al.* (2016), in so far as closeness to dementia affects understanding and priorities, but in complex ways, mediated by age, that need further exploration. What we have been able to add to the debate is a concern with generational priorities in exploring how more meaningful, age-tailored messages can be achieved to enhance understanding across age groups in relation to dementia.

The possibility of increased understanding through recognising othering as a social, age-related phenomenon presents novel challenges to public health interventions related to dementia. Embedding attitudes to dementia within attitudes to adult ageing, creates the possibility that understanding is doubly othered, making empathic understanding between age groups particularly difficult. Whilst a focus on prevention is desirable, an emphasis on the fact that dementia is a pathological condition rather than a normal part of ageing may further complicate the task of empathic understanding. For while it has proven useful for awareness-raising and has helped in distancing an enduring self from the condition, it compromises the connective value of the realisation that, if we are lucky enough, 'we all grow old'. By contrast, recognising memory loss as a common experience across age groups might reduce othering. Different age groups may have specific motivations to perceive dementia as relatively normal or as a disease process other than the self, making these dynamics complex and requiring further qualitative study.

How, then, might dementia as the radically 'not me' engage with a 'me in the future' as intimated by adult ageing? Conceptually speaking, this radical distancing requires a radical repositioning of othering in relation to the self. Positive othering, for example, constitutes insightful consideration of distinctiveness based on adult age, where difference is valued in the process of establishing genuine and respectful encounters (Biggs 2018). Once the distinctive positions of the protagonists are recognised and given voice, it is then possible to begin a process of realistic understanding, based on the actual rather than assumed positions of the age-other. It allows the complementary nature of relationships and empathic understanding of the other to emerge.

A renewed focus on positive othering, which recognises differences as well as commonalities between age groups and phenomena associated with age, may help recognition and valorising of ageing, disease and associated experiences. This would form a first step to bridging the divides between categories which may currently be inhibiting the adoption of public health messages and ultimately social adaptation to dementia.

Differences emerged in our study, not only between age-groups' own responses but also in between their own and the views thought to be held by particular age groups in the public domain. This raises interesting issues regarding mismatch between the actual perceptions of age groups and the attribution of views supposedly held in the public sphere. Possible game changers are reflected in the importance attributed to personal contact with dementia; and, in older groups, the focus on communication and practical understanding. A generational intelligence approach indicates that positive personal contact might succeed in enhancing emotional and cognitive connections to dementia. Interaction with people living with dementia or their families was the most frequently cited reason for people to positively encounter dementia, even though it was also cited as something the general public avoided.

Recognising differences between the attitudes and priorities of particular age groups will also help to critically address understanding between people with dementia and others, a factor that will become increasingly important if alliances are to be made in the shift from a medical to a social understanding of dementia (Swaffer 2015).

While current public health interventions are commonly designed without consumer participation, they are becoming increasingly challenged as dementia activists insist that their voice be heard and distinctions made between professional voice and the voice of people living with or affected by dementia (Bartlett 2017). We argue that when the specific experience and circumstances of people with dementia and their care/support partners is recognised, age should also play a major part in designing future public health campaigns and interventions.

This study of the relationship between attitudes towards ageing, perceptions of dementia and the age of the receiver demonstrates that the age of the perceiver is an important factor in assessing attitudes towards dementia. What is significant is that attitudes towards ageing and dementia interact in ways that may influence the reception of public health messaging, with positive understanding being enhanced by greater contact. An approach needs to be developed that values the distinctiveness of each age-groups' position in respect to dementia, as a foundation for positive understanding and solidarity to emerge.

## Note

1 The project is funded through the National Health and Medical Research Council Cognitive Decline Partnership Centre (http://sydney.edu.au/medicine/cdpc/) and partners, ethical approval number HESC 1647136.

## References

Australian Census, 2011, *Australian Census of Population and Housing*, www.abs.gov.au/ausstats/abs@.nsf/Lookup/2071.0main+features902012-2013.

Alzheimer Europe, 2011, Value of knowing: Report of key findings Five-Country Alzheimer's Disease Survey, *Harvard School of Public Health and Alzheimer Europe*, www.alzheimer-europe.org/Research/Value-of-Knowing.

Au, A., S. Biggs, S-T. Cheng, I. Haapala, D. Gallagher-Thompson, (in press), Connecting through caregiving in dementia: Reappraisal via perspective-taking on intergenerational relationships, *Research in Social Work Practice*.

Ballenger, J.F., 2006, The biomedical deconstruction of senility and the persistent stigmatization of old age in the United States, in A. Leibing and L. Cohen (eds), *Thinking About Dementia: Culture, Loss, and the Anthropology of Senility*, pp. 106–120, New Brunswick, USA: Rutgers University Press.

Bartlett, R., 2017, Suffering with dementia: The other side of 'living well', *International Psychogeriatrics*, 29(2): 177–179.

Behuniak, S., 2011, The living dead?: The construction of people with Alzheimer's disease as zombies, *Ageing and Society*, 31(01): 70–92.

Bernasconi, R., 2012, Othering, in F. Halsall, J. Jansen, S. Murphy (eds), *Critical Communities and Aesthetic Practices: Contributions to Phenomenology*, Volume 64, pp. 151–157, Dordrecht, The Netherlands: Springer.

Biggs, S., 2018, *Negotiating Ageing: Cultural Adaptation to the Prospect of a Long Life*, London: Routledge.

Biggs, S., A. Lowenstein, 2011, *Generational Intelligence: A Critical Approach to Age Relations*, New York: Routledge.

Biggs, S., I. Haapala, A. Lowenstein, 2011, Exploring generational intelligence as a model for examining the process of intergenerational relationships, *Ageing and Society*, 31(7): 1107–1124.

Bollas, C., 1989, *Forces of Destiny: Psychoanalysis and Human Idiom*, London: Free Association Books.

Brownson, R.C., R.G. Tabak, K.A. Stamatakis, K. Glanz, 2015, Implementation, dissemination and diffusion of public health interventions, in K. Glanz, B.K. Rimer, K. Viswanath (eds), *Health Behavior: Theory, Research, and Practice*, Fifth edition, pp. 301–326, San Francisco, USA: Jossey-Bass.

Cahill, S., M. Pierce, P. Werner, A. Darley, A. Bobersky, 2015, A systematic review of the public's knowledge and understanding of Alzheimer's disease and dementia, *Alzheimer Disease and Associated Disorders*, 29(3): 255–275.

Cheston, R., J. Hancock, and P. White, 2016, A cross-sectional investigation of public attitudes toward dementia in Bristol and South Gloucestershire using the approaches to dementia questionnaire, *International Psychogeriatrics*, 28(10): 1717–1724.

Dow, B., M. Joosten, S. Biggs, H. Kimberley, 2016, Age encounters: Exploring age and intergenerational perceptions, *Journal of Intergenerational Relationships*, 14(2): 104–118.

Gerritsen, D.L., J. Oyebode, D. Gove, 2016, Ethical implications of the perception and portrayal of dementia, *Dementia*, 0(0): 1-13.

Glynn, R., Shelley, E., B. Lawlor, 2017, Public knowledge and understanding of dementia: Evidence from a national survey in Ireland, *Age and ageing*, 46(5): 865–869.

Grattan Institute, 2014, *The Wealth of Generations*, https://grattan.edu.au/report/the-wealth-of-generations/ [Accessed 20 October 2017].

Haapala, I., A. Carr, S. Biggs, (in press), What would I want: Dementia perspectives and priorities? *International Journal of Care and Caring*.

Haapala, I., L. Tervo, S. Biggs, 2015, Using generational intelligence to examine community care work between younger and older adults, *Journal of Social Work Practice*, 29(4): 457–473.

Intergenerational Foundation, 2015, *Intergenerational Fairness Index*, www.if.org.uk/archives/6909/2015-intergenerational-fairness-index [Accessed 06 December 2015].

Kivipelto, M., F. Mangialasche, T. Ngandu, 2017, Can lifestyle changes prevent cognitive impairment?, *The Lancet Neurology*, 16(5): 338–339.

Kohli, M., 2005, Generational changes and generational equity, in M.L. Johnson (ed.), *The Cambridge Handbook of Age and Ageing*, pp. 518–526, Cambridge, UK: Cambridge University Press.

Léon, C., S. Pin, C. Kreft-Jais, P. Arwidson, 2015, Perceptions of Alzheimer's disease in the French population, *Journal of Alzheimer's Disease*, 47: 467–478.

Livingston, G., A. Sommerlad, V. Orgeta, S.G. Costafreda, J. Huntley, D. Ames, C. Ballard, S. Banerjee, A. Burns, J. Cohen-Mansfield, C. Cooper, 2017, Dementia prevention, intervention, and care, *The Lancet*, 390(10113): 2673–2734.

Marshall, V.W., 2007, Advancing the sociology of ageism, *Social Forces*, 86(1): 257–264.

Minkler, M., A. Robertson, 1991, The ideology of age-race wars, *Ageing and Society*, 11(1): 1–22.

Moody, H.R., 2008, Aging America and the boomer wars, *The Gerontologist*, 48(6): 839–844.

Phillips, J.E., K.J. Ajrouch, S. Hillcoat-Nallétamby, 2010, *Key Concepts in Social Gerontology*, Los Angeles, USA: Sage.

Phillipson, L., D.C. Magee, S. Jones, D.E. Kladzien, 2014, Correlates of dementia attitudes in a sample of middle-aged Australian adults, *Australasian Journal on Ageing*, 33(3): 158–163.

Prince, M., 2017, Progress on dementia: Leaving no one behind, *The Lancet*, 390(10113): E51-E53.

Prince, M., A. Wimo, M. Guerchet, G.C. Ali, Y.T. Wu, M. Prina, *World Alzheimer Report 2015, The Global Impact of Dementia: An Analysis of Prevalence, Incidence, Cost and Trends*, London: Alzheimer's Disease International.

Scodellaro, C., S. Pin, 2013, The ambiguous relationships between ageing and Alzheimer's disease: A critical literature review, *Dementia*, 12(1): 137–151.

Smith, B.J., S. Ali, H. Quach, 2014, Public knowledge and beliefs about dementia risk reduction: A national survey of Australians, *BMC Public Health*, 14(1): 1.

Swaffer, K., 2015, *Dementia and Prescribed Disengagement™*, London: Sage Publications.

Van Gorp, B., T. Vercruysse, J. Van den Bulck, 2012, Toward a more nuanced perception of Alzheimer's disease: Designing and testing a campaign advertisement, *American Journal of Alzheimer's Disease & Other Dementias*, 27(6): 388–396.

World Health Organization, 2012, *Dementia: A Public Health Priority*, Geneva, Switzerland: World Health Organization, www.who.int/mental_health/publications/dementia_report_2012/en/.

World Health Organization, 2016, *WHO Global Action Plan on the Public Health Response to Dementia 2017–2025* (EB140/28), Geneva, Switzerland: World Health Organisation, www.who.int/mental_health/neurology/dementia/action_plan_consultation/en/.

Williamson, J.B., T.K. McNamara, S.A. Howling, 2003, Generational equity, generational interdependence, and the framing of the debate over social security reform, *Journal of Sociology and Social Welfare*, 30(3): 3–14.

Winblad, B., P. Amouyel, S. Andrieu, C. Ballard, C. Brayne, H. Brodaty, H. Feldman, 2016, Defeating Alzheimer's disease and other dementias: A priority for European science and society, *The Lancet Neurology*, 15(5): 455–532.

Zelig, H., 2014, Dementia as a cultural metaphor, *The Gerontologist*, 54(2): 258–267.

# Part II
# Autonomy and dignity

# 6 Developing a relational approach to decision-making in healthcare settings

*Suzanne Jarrad*

In this chapter, decision-making, as a central component of personal autonomy, is explored through a case study of the kinds of decision-making processes used with vulnerable older people in a healthcare setting. Andrei's story illustrates that the assumptions made by professionals about the lack of decision-making abilities of older people who display symptoms of cognitive impairment lead to practices that further reduce autonomy, and thus social personhood. I identify current approaches that contribute to negative outcomes for people such as Andrei, and propose an approach for use in healthcare settings that recognises the relational aspects of autonomy, and facilitates participation of the older person in decision-making about their own lives to the fullest extent possible.

## Introduction

In the liberal model of autonomy, a person who is regarded as legally or socially autonomous is given personhood status, along with accompanying rights. In this way, personhood is understood as a status bestowed on others, and is linked to the value given to specific attributes, which might vary in any given social and cultural context (Naffine 2009: 10). In the western tradition, the most dominant personhood attribute has come to be that of the rational thinking individual (Naffine 2009). This has emerged from the values of liberalism: the ideal of citizens having the liberty to self-govern, free to choose their own authentic 'good' without interference by others (Mill 1906; Rawls 1971; Kukathas 1993). This understanding of autonomy, as a form of self-government, requires the cognitive ability to reason, as an internal process of critical reflection and evaluation (Agich 1990). In this view, autonomy is absolute – either one has it or one does not. Those without this substantive ability are considered unable to be self-determining. Consequently, their social status is devalued and they join a lesser class of persons, such as children and those with mental illness, who reside on the 'margins' of personhood and law (Carney 1991).

There are many powerful critiques pointing to the limitations of the liberal ideal of reason. Nevertheless, it is a foundational ideology, and tenacious. It assumes each citizen possesses equal abilities and attributes, whereas in reality, people vary in abilities and attributes (Stone 1991), and liberalism ignores many of these differences. Other critiques include the fact that the ability to reason is assessed in terms of a culturally-laden continuum. There is no such thing as a fully achievable rational ability; even what is seen as rational, non-rational or irrational is culturally specific, inflected by, for example, class, age and gender. This makes the establishment of a clear threshold for autonomy problematic (Narayan 2002; Christman 2003; Stoljar 2013).

From a moral perspective, the exclusive nature of the liberal notion of autonomy denies full personhood status to those who do not meet a rational cognitive ideal. Post (1995, 2006: 224) describes the consequent differentiation of human worth as producing elitism in this 'hyper-cognitive' society.

Another concern arising from the liberal emphasis on the attribute of reason is that it ignores the essential contribution of values, emotions and intuition in enabling individuals to determine personal priorities in decision-making (Charland 1998; Devereaux and Parker 2006). Evidence from neuroscience supports a view that human beings are not predominantly rational. For example, neural pathways of 'fast' and 'slow' thinking indicate that humans often use fast intuitive thinking rather than reasoning in day-to-day functioning and decision-making, and more so when they are older (Wood and Tanius 2007).

Despite these criticisms, the liberal ideal of reason as a dominant attribute of personhood is pervasive in western society. The liberal paradigm is utilised in legal approaches, such as common law approaches to legal capacity. This framework becomes especially contentious when it is used to remove decision-making rights unnecessarily or inappropriately.

This chapter discusses case studies regarding the adequacy of recognition of older peoples' autonomy in decision-making. It draws on a relational understanding of personhood so as to develop a more appropriate model for relational decision-making that avoids paternalism, moving the focus from the expertise and authority of health professionals to a relationship with the patient based on respect and empathy.

## Personhood, autonomy and dementia

The construct of human worth as based on cognitive ability significantly shapes attitudes towards those with neurocognitive disorders such as dementia. In surveys reported by Alzheimer's Australia in 2011, 63 per cent of Australians were more afraid of getting dementia than any other health condition. There is evidence of social avoidance, with 22 per cent saying they would 'feel uncomfortable spending time with someone with dementia' (Alzheimer's Australia 2011: 4). Shame, humiliation and fear are reported as reactions when people are confronted with the scenario of being diagnosed with a form of dementia themselves (Phillipson *et al.* 2012: 9).

Because our value and status as a person is socially constructed in complex ways, any form of stigma has a strong undermining effect on us. Stigma results in the person being 'reduced in our minds from a whole and usual person to a tainted, discounted one' (Goffman 1961: 12), which leads to 'sympathy, pity or invasive paternalism' (Christman 2003: 3). The fear and stigma associated with dementia means that stereotypes about the inability of someone with dementia to make decisions contribute to attitudes and practices that, in turn, act to confirm preconceived assumptions of incapacity (cf. Phillipson *et al.* 2012: 10). For example, one study on the decision-making of persons in early stage dementia found that people's opinions were 'often overlooked and their rights to information and free expression [were] fragile' (Tyrrell *et al.* 2006: 496). Labels such as 'lacking insight' are judgemental and thus they become depersonalising and reduce a person's sense of identity. They affect dignity, independence and the recognition of rights (Bond *et al.* 2002: 313) long before advanced cognitive decline makes a person truly incapable.

There has been increasing medicalisation of dementia over the past two decades, with dominance given to biomedical understandings (Lyman 1989; Bond 1992; Macdonald 2018). While there have been benefits to people with dementia and their families through the medical legitimation of the condition, this trend has reduced the social status of those with a diagnosis of dementia because it focuses on anticipated deficits, rather than the possibilities for living a full life through a range of abilities (Bond 1992). Behuniak (2011: 85–86) argues that the focus on the most demeaning of the symptoms of dementia, and the 'destructive representation' of a person with dementia as the 'living dead', exacerbates fear and destroys empathy and respect.

It was Kitwood who first challenged the reductionist biomedical model and the limited social construction of personhood in dementia, with a view of personhood as relational, occurring 'in the context of relationship and social being' (1997: 8). He developed the phrase 'malignant social psychology' to identify attitudes and practices that affected the identity and self-esteem of people with dementia, and reduced their worth as persons (1997: 45). Importantly, he also identified how a negative social and psychological environment could compound the symptoms of dementia, indicating the profound importance of environments that support and nurture persons (Kitwood 1997). This provides a clear understanding of people experiencing dementia as continuing to be responsive to relationships and social contexts. The impact of negativity is similar in effect to that of ageism, which also gives rise to stereotypes and paternalism, and is experienced as demeaning by those targeted.

## Ageism, cognition and personhood

While there has been increasing incidence of the diagnosis of younger people with dementia, the majority (over 90 per cent) are in later life, over the age of 65 years (Alzheimer Australia 2017). Older people already experience diminished social status and prejudice from ageism and this is further challenged in the diminishing of social value that accompanies cognitive changes. There is a two-way effect in play: older persons are subjected to ageist assumptions made about their cognitive ability, on the basis of common age-related changes (such as slower recall, vulnerability to short-term confusion), and when these are assumed to be symptoms of dementia, they result in further stigmatisation. Older people often report being treated as if they are incompetent, impassive and incapable of decision-making, and are thus excluded from opportunities to participate (Cuddy and Fiske 2004; Batsch and Mittleman 2012; Australian Law Reform Commission 2017).

A major issue arising from prescribed social roles and labels is the tendency for an older person to internalise them, consequently reducing their sense of self-respect and self-worth (Benson 1994; McLeod 2002). This can shape the older person's behaviour in a process of 'behavioural confirmation' (Cuddy and Fiske 2004; Kite and Wagner 2004: 18), leading to 'excess disability' (Power 2014: 140). These patterns also get internalised into approaches to care.

Societal stereotypes about older persons and ageist attitudes can become 'imbedded in care systems' (Surtees 2014: 453). Health professionals are 'as likely to be prejudiced against older people as other individuals' (Lothian and Philp 2001; Nelson 2005: 211) and are 'a major source of ageist treatment' (Minichello *et al.* 2000: 253). This can include limiting information and choices (Resnick *et al.* 1998; Kite and Wagner 2004). Older people become vulnerable to these norms and power imbalances.

One risk of such imbalances is undue paternalism towards those who are considered 'lesser' in social terms (Christman 2003). Paternalism is evident when someone deliberately exerts power over another to impose restrictions on that person's liberty or autonomy, on the assumption (based on perceptions, beliefs or some other rationale) that they are providing a benefit to the person (Kleinig 1983). Strong paternalism occurs when the will of a competent person is overridden, weak paternalism is intervention on behalf of those who are not considered competent and whose choices may carry a risk of harm (Kerridge *et al.* 1998). Both rely on a moral justification that the action taken is beneficial to the person, is in their best interests and is catering to 'the welfare, good, happiness, needs, interests or values of the person' (Dworkin 1971: 108).

Paternalism is underpinned by the belief or assertion that the person concerned has a poor ability to know what is best for them, and that their own choices will result in poor outcomes. This includes an implicit moral judgement by others about the person's inability to 'pursue their own good' (Christman 2003: 9), with the belief that one has greater knowledge as to what another's 'good' is. Whether strong or weak, paternalism is detrimental, depriving a person of their right or capacity to act. It can also be the case that a decision-maker has an incomplete or distorted knowledge of a person, and has filtered information through their own values and preferences (Kleinig 1983); or made decisions 'in haste, [or] driven by resource issues' (Bigby *et al.* 2015: 5). Paternalistic practices lead to the loss of available options, limiting choice, and leading to possibly unanticipated or unwanted outcomes (Stoljar 2013: 5).

Weak paternalism, as decision-making and intervention on behalf of a person considered to lack capacity, has traditionally been accepted as justified if it protects a person from harm (Faden *et al.* 1986; Carney 1991; Devereaux and Parker 2006). This paternalism is sufficiently evident and problematic that it is now challenged through human rights frameworks. The United Nations Convention on the Rights of Persons with Disabilities asserts in Article 12 that persons with disabilities have the right to participate in decisions and be provided with support to do so (United Nations 2006). This has resulted in changes in policy and practice in the disability sector towards support for self-determination (Bigby *et al.* 2015). However, dementia still sits in an ambiguous space, not defined as a disability under Australia's National Disability Insurance Scheme, except in some cases of younger onset.

The Australian Law Reform Commission, in reviewing Australian law in response to these concerns, has also affirmed the importance of upholding the individual autonomy of older persons undergoing cognitive changes:

> the right to enjoy a self-determined life is particularly important in consideration of older persons with impaired or declining cognitive abilities. It reflects the paradigm shift towards supported decision making … so that it is the will and preferences of the person that drives decisions.
>
> (2017: 1.104)

These principles challenge the reduced social status of those treated as 'lesser' persons due to cognitive disability, arguing for a new paradigm that gives focus to the person's voice in decision-making, to the extent it is possible. In giving primary respect to the person's own conception of 'good', autonomy is recognised as an intrinsic human need and a source of motivation for living (Deci 1980), increasing wellbeing and quality of life (Brown and Brown 2009). There is increasing acknowledgement of the harm to self-esteem and self-identity that occurs when overriding the will of another, with the resulting sense of powerlessness and hopelessness (Winick 1996; Woolhead *et al.* 2004; Stoljar 2013).

Respect for autonomy is a challenging concept to apply in the face of progressive cognitive impairment such as dementia. In the broadest sense, to act in a self-determining way is understood to be the expression of a person's internal thoughts, values and emotions, which comprise their unique sense of self in response to their exterior world. Respect for autonomy lies in enabling their voice to be heard and their underlying values need to be interpreted within the knowledge of the person's history, life meaning and current experience of reality. This connects to the concept of relationality, where social and personal relationships shape the person's sense of self and their adaptation to their changing world.

## A relational approach towards personhood and dementia

A relational approach towards people with dementia gives recognition to the constitutive elements of social relationships, with the understanding that participation in decision-making, important to wellbeing, can be facilitated or inhibited by others. This relational foundation is given expression in the human rights call for support in decision-making for those with disabilities, acknowledging the importance of affirmative activities to enhance individual capacity to participate in decisions about their lives.

The relational approach is underpinned by a broader view of the person with dementia beyond the medicalised focus on cognitive deficits, recognising personal attributes such as 'autonomy, social and cognitive abilities, an intact sense of social and personal identity, humour and individuality, and agency and the capacity to value' (Epp 2003: 15). Rather than brain changes defining the person with dementia, there is respect for the person's emotions, intuition, will and sense of self: a 'valuer' rather than a 'cogniser' (Jaworska 1999: 130).

Symptoms that had previously been considered to result solely from neuropathological damage have instead been identified as resulting from the interactions between personality, biography, physical health, neurologic impairment and social psychology (Epp 2003). For example, agitation, often a symptom related to dementia, can be due to undiagnosed pain, or excessive noise and stimulation. In an ideal situation of appropriate psychological support, people with dementia can experience improved cognitive functioning and adapt to their environment (Kitwood and Benson 1995; Woods and Pratt 2005; Bredesen 2014). The person's ability to express their autonomy, shaped by these attributes of the self, can also be supported or diminished by their social environment and relationships (O'Connor and Purves 2009).

At the frontier of the application of the new paradigm about dementia is the deconstruction of preconceptions arising from the biomedical view. A focus on pathology is instead replaced by a focus on the whole person, who is living and adapting to the disease, and using language to describe these effects that is 'as free of judgement and stigma as possible' (Power 2014: 19). This includes recognising that persons with dementia have shifting cognitive pathways that utilise feelings and symbols instead of or in addition to memories and facts, and have increased awareness of emotional environments (Power 2014: 19). This relational approach, based on empathy and imbedded within relationships, broadens the recognition of other attributes of the person with dementia that affect the status bestowed by others.

A number of personal narratives by people living with dementia have provided a greater understanding of their subjective experiences of their symptoms, their increasing dependency on others and the stigma and assumptions they encounter which further disable them personally and socially (Taylor 2007; Bryden 2012; Swaffer 2014). There is increased recognition that the person with dementia is the best 'expert' on themselves, reflected in their increasing involvement in the decisions affecting their lives (Brooker 2004). Inclusive practices previously denied the diagnosed person, are slowly being incorporated into practice. These include informing people of their diagnosis (Maguire *et al.* 1996); enabling participation in feedback about services (Epp 2003); empowering them with knowledge about how to live with the disease (Alzheimer's Australia 2014); and educating others as to the lived experience of dementia (Swaffer 2014).

In recognising that all of us navigate life through various challenges, and make adaptations in response, a counter-narrative to dementia views it not as a 'catastrophic model' but a 'biographical disruption', requiring adjustment, accommodation and reconciliation (Clarke *et al.* 2011: 14–15). The experience and wellbeing of the person becomes the primary focus, rather than a focus on brain pathology and its effects. Symptoms are understood as expressions of the person's lack of psychological and physical wellbeing, rather than solely the effect of organic brain changes. Power suggests that focusing on the whole person transforms understanding, from the traditional view of loss of self to an understanding that the person with dementia is experiencing their disability as the 'new normal', opening up the possibilities of enhancing functioning through 'strength-based approaches' (2014: 22–23). For Power (2014), this translates to shaping the care environment and developing a culture which, rather than measuring medical outcomes and levels of functioning, focuses on aspects of wellbeing for each individual. Learning the strengths and abilities of each person provides practical opportunities to respond to needs in wellbeing domains such as identity, connectedness, security, autonomy and meaning.

This wellbeing approach supports the need for the provision of supportive social environments that acknowledge and respond to emotion, and nurture the person's abilities and skills (Kitwood 1997). Other approaches towards care include recognising that each person has a unique history and worldview, focusing on a person's strengths and abilities, ensuring choice, supporting their decision-making, 'providing unconditional positive regard' (Nay *et al.* 2009: 110) and 'an environment that is always ... conducive to the articulation of one's unique personhood' (Davis 2004: 376). This implementation of these principles into practice are challenging, but have already contributed towards changes in some settings where the care approach does not give priority to functional care tasks and 'doing to', but instead to one where relationships based on wellbeing and empowerment are central (Brooker 2004; Loveday 2013; Power 2014).

Philosophically and socially, recognising that the human experience of value and wellbeing extends well beyond the attribute of cognition, challenges the rationalist model. Instead of being static and absolute, autonomy is more realistically understood as a dynamic and changing state, developed from birth and shaped throughout life within the context of relationships, requiring an understanding of the variable influences in real life that are constitutive of autonomy (Nedelsky 2011). For those living with dementia, their experience of the day-to-day, their sense of self and their autonomy and capacity for decision-making, can all be enhanced or diminished by the attitudes and behaviour of those around them. From this theoretical base, I undertook a study to explore how decision-making was taking place in practice in relation to vulnerable older people.

## The research: personhood in the healthcare setting

The healthcare environment of the hospital was selected as one most likely to raise issues around decision-making, and one in which older persons constitute a high percentage of patients. I utilised a case study approach to enable detailed exploration of decision-making within a complex environment. Six cases were recruited, where the older person was over the age of 65 years, and at the point when they were being assessed for decision-making capacity.[1]

Data was gathered from multiple sources, including my observations and field notes of the assessment for capacity, my interviews with the assessor and family members and from comprehensive field notes made from the case file. This included admission reports, professional assessments and reports and progress notes by health professionals throughout the admission. Particular attention was given to evidence of decisions made and by whom, and any recorded viewpoint of the older person. The older person was not interviewed directly due to ethical issues of consent, and I looked to interpret their perspective where possible from the data collected.

Each type of data was transposed into text with each case participant given a pseudonym. Nuanced information came from analysing the text for themes and using filters such as knowledge about the person; expressed attitudes towards the older person; expressed personal and professional values; hospital processes; the language and views of doctors and allied health staff in the case file; evidence for cognitive impairment; and the interpretation of law regarding decision-making capacity.

The case studies focused on four men and two women, ranging in age from 77 years to 89 years. Four were living in their own home prior to hospital admission, and two in supported accommodation. One person was admitted due to an inability to cope at home, and three were admitted following a fall. Behaviour changes creating a crisis in living situation was the reason for the remaining two admissions. All but one person had experienced age-related physical decline in the year prior to admission, with one person particularly frail from the combination of an earlier adverse medical event, surgery and the effects of a terminal respiratory illness.

Only two of the six case subjects had a clinical diagnosis of dementia; with five of the six experiencing temporary confusion during their hospital stay. From the five capacity assessments conducted, two of the persons were found to be capable and three as not having capacity to make the decision in question. The voice and personhood of the older person was found to be diminished in the hospital setting, constraining options and participation in decision-making about their lives. Four of the subjects were admitted to an aged care residential facility, and all were reluctant. A fifth person resisted pressure to enter a residential facility and returned home on trial before being admitted to another hospital and dying several weeks later. The option of residential care was raised by a social worker during a confessional episode of the person in the sixth case, but was not pursued when the person improved cognitively.

### Case study: Andrei

I elaborate the case of Andrei to illustrate a number of these elements before returning to a more general discussion of the case study findings. I begin with Andrei's background and the events leading up to admission as provided by his son and daughter-in-law in interview, and then continue the story of his hospital experience chronologically, as developed from his hospital file.

Andrei, aged 87, was born in East Prussia, and immigrated to Australia in early adulthood with his wife and son. At the time of the study, he had been living alone in the family home for three decades and, as a result of glaucoma, had lost his sight six months earlier. Andrei's son and daughter-in-law had been providing daily meals, and the district nurse visited for daily medication checks and weekly hygiene assistance. There had been no apparent specialist support for Andrei to deal with his blindness, during or following his full loss of sight. Andrei had been on a waiting list for home care services for 12 months. Since experiencing total blindness, he was reported as being frequently frustrated and irritable. His daughter-in-law was experiencing stress in providing constant meals, and finding Andrei to be increasingly demanding and lacking any apparent appreciation of her help. Andrei had lapsed at times into speaking German, and experienced vivid 'dreams' at times, signs the family saw of changing cognition. A few weeks prior to his hospital admission, Andrei increasingly complained of constipation, and on one visit, his daughter-in-law found faeces on the doorframes and handles of the house. When this occurred several more times, she refused to assist with his care, and the GP recommended that Andrei be taken to hospital, where he was admitted for 'failure to cope'.

From Andrei's point of view, the total loss of vision was difficult and had a profound effect on his day-to-day lived experience. Indeed, he reported to his son that, as his sight deteriorated, day and night became blurred, and he was unable to carry out his usual activities, such as cooking. He told his son about having vivid daytime 'dreams' which made discerning reality difficult at times. Time dragged, with an occasional visit by the District Nurse, a brief evening visit by his daughter-in-law with his home cooked meal and weekend visits by his son. He reports becoming increasingly uncomfortable with daily constipation, which may have been caused by dehydration or poor diet, and although an X-ray organised by his GP revealed nothing untoward, the problem continued and he sought relief through manual means. He could not see the mess he was making. With his daughter-in-law's reaction in withdrawing daily assistance and his GP's recommendation, Andrei agreed to be taken to hospital.

The first phase of analysis was of the language used in the case file. The case notes by each health professional was converted to text, and words used to describe Andrei were analysed and numbered if indicative of deficits or assets. The results suggested a distinctive framing of Andrei's attributes as a person, starting at admission. For example, deficit language recorded in the case file by the admitting doctor emphasised illness and dependency, shaping Andrei's recorded identity: disoriented; general decline; failure to cope: situational crisis; early dementia; and obsessed with bowel movements [sic]. Some of the wording implied judgements rather than observations, such as 'obsessed'. The asset words recorded by the admitting doctor mainly gave facts on Andrei's background, such as: former cabinet maker; lives alone in house he built 60 years ago; and very supportive family. These were less frequent in number when compared with deficit words.

Following admission and during the first three and a half days in hospital, Andrei was seen by the Medical Registrar, the Resident Medical Officer, the Medical Consultant and team on a ward round, an occupational therapist, a speech pathologist and a social worker, each of whom recorded their professional views and assessment in the case file.

The content of these notes reflected the role of each professional. For instance, the Registrar, from his medical review, recorded 'functional decline culminating in an episode at home where he had been worried about constipation, attempted manual evacuation and was found by family with faeces spread everywhere', and 'underlying dementia'. The nursing staff, who made regular notes in the file, reported that Andrei had some 'periods of agitation' which seemed to 'settle after the first few days' when his sleeping improved. The occupational therapist noted in her assessment that it was questionable as to whether 'Andrei had full insight into the support required by family for him to stay at home'. The physiotherapist recorded that the family could no longer provide the care required. Overall, these assessments contributed to the picture of Andrei as experiencing functional physical and cognitive decline, with questionable insight into the support required to live at home and his family members experiencing strain in providing care.

There was an absence of any report regarding an assessment or diagnosis of Andrei's cognitive status, or exclusionary tests, and, therefore, a lack of evidence of cognitive impairment. The issue of constipation was not apparent in the clinical notes, suggesting that it had resolved. There were no clinical notes as to the effect of his blindness in an unfamiliar environment, or of resources that could further support him. There was no evidence in the notes that Andrei had been asked about what he thought he might need to stay at home.

From the 'problem', as recorded by a range of professional perspectives, the healthcare team devised the 'solution' of residential care, which was followed by a case conference with members of the healthcare team and immediate family, but which excluded Andrei. In response to concern by the son that Andrei might change his mind about accepting residential care, the social worker referred Andrei for a capacity assessment, and also suggested an application to the Guardianship Board, which the son understood would lead to his appointment as a substitute decision-maker in the event that Andrei resisted the option of residential care. The proposed outcome of entering residential care was communicated to Andrei, who was then given time to think about this news, give assent and be involved in participating in the choice of facility, demonstrating a strong paternalistic approach.

Following the referral for a capacity assessment, the Consultant overseeing the case assessed Andrei and made a determination of capacity to make a decision about his accommodation, based on having insight into his care needs:

> [he] recognised … his vision limited his ability to remain at home … so personally I was surprised that capacity was even raised … because he had insight into his medical problems and appropriately assessed that he needed some more help.

The Consultant noted that Andrei 'was also willing to go to more supportive care'. However, analysis of the dialogue in the assessment interview demonstrated a distinct bias on the part of the Consultant as to the benefits of residential care for Andrei. The Consultant did not facilitate a discussion on understanding alternative options, and was not neutral to the outcome of the decision. Instead he directed the interview to the desirability of residential care, ignoring and overriding Andrei's expressed preference:

ANDREI: But I don't want to leave home.
CONSULTANT: But you would get more help.

Significantly, the finding of a decision-making capacity did not activate an alternative response that respected Andrei's autonomy, nor did Andrei receive any further advice on options or support for his preferences. His family were in agreement with the proposal of residential aged care, and with the lack of any supportive voice, when a vacancy arose at a preferred aged care facility, Andrei was transferred there from hospital. In this situation, Andrei had little agency, and seemingly no choice but to comply.

Assumptions regarding Andrei's cognition were evident. A query about early dementia was noted at the time of admission, with the Registrar noting 'underlying dementia', and stating the possibility of Andrei having Lewy Body type dementia, based on the reported hallucinations. An alternative explanation for these was that of brain responses to the sensory deprivation of blindness (see Kester 2009). Similarly, his agitation and confusion in hospital may have been a result of short-term delirium due to medication. These assumptions were not tested clinically and shaped the approach by the allied health professionals. For example, Andrei was not given the opportunity to make his own decision about his care and accommodation, and was referred for a capacity assessment as lacking insight into his care needs. An application to the Guardianship Board for a substitute decision-maker reinforces this assumption, with the social worker advising the son that this would enable him to become the legal decision-maker and thus be able to ensure the outcome of residential care.

Notably, the view of the Consultant that Andrei had a legal capacity to decide his care and accommodation did not trigger a change of approach on the part of the healthcare team, which would have been evidenced by them respecting Andrei's expressed preference to return home. The focus instead was on achieving the planned solution, not on respecting autonomy. Overall, the assumption of the presence of dementia became conflated with decision-making incapacity, which led to paternalistic and exclusionary practices in decision-making.

While the son and daughter-in-law had previously provided assistance to Andrei to continue living at home, in their interview they indicated their lack of support for Andrei to stay at home any longer. Andrei had refused earlier suggestions of care from his son, and the incident with the faeces became a trigger for admission, with willingness by the son for the hospital to facilitate the solution of residential care. The family's care burden was given greater weight than

Andrei's preferences, rather than exploration and negotiation of a solution that recognised the autonomy and needs of both Andrei and his family members. The hospital became a place of negotiation and brokering of personal life solutions beyond the scope of medical assessment and treatment, with accompanying bio-medical values dominating rather than those reflecting social personhood.

Based on the information gained from the interviews and the files, Andrei's past experience of living alone and more recently, his ability to manage his basic activities of daily living at home, despite his visual impairment and with only the assistance of meals and medications, was given no recognition. The importance of Andrei's familiar environment in maximising his day-to-day independence was also not acknowledged. There was no stated or recorded consideration of other resources that might support his preference to return home, such as pursuing his eligibility for a high care package at home to assist with hygiene and meals, and support and respite for family members. Alternative options that may have worked for all parties were not explored. A 'protective' solution, clearly not in his best interests, was imposed on Andrei, and his preference was not given serious consideration. Andrei was subjected to reduced moral and legal status and, with the resultant powerlessness, he was given no choice and was unable to assert his preference.

This outcome could have been different if there had been greater recognition of Andrei's needs and respect for his preferences. A relational response to Andrei's home situation prior to hospital admission would have been for family and healthcare providers to appreciate his strong wish to continue residing at home, and to recognise the significant benefits for Andrei, now blind, because he knew his home's physical environment. Greater attention would have been paid to his physical comfort and managing the symptoms of constipation, through providing Andrei with information about the common causes, and engaging him in considering options such as increased fluids, dietary changes or pharmacy products and offering monitoring support by the District Nursing service.

Discussing the requirement for sustainable cultural-appropriate meals with Andrei, and options for other sources of meals and their costs, could have led to a better independent arrangement, and significantly reduced the stress and nega-tivity experienced by his daughter-in-law. Involving Andrei in these issues and their solutions would have been empowering for him and would have supported his autonomy.

The outcome also could have been different in hospital if Andrei had had someone advocating on his behalf, such as a social worker. Such support could have enabled exploration of other solutions that could have relieved the family of care tasks while enabling Andrei to return home.

### The case study themes

The case study approach, with its multiple perspectives, enables in-depth exploration and analysis of an issue. The six case studies all provided nuanced examples of how the dynamics of social relationships, power differentials, cultural norms and prevailing values, affected the autonomy of the vulnerable older person in the hospital setting.

Medicine, with its social and scientific authority, is dominant in such settings, with a focus on disease, and the doctor as expert. These norms shape the views and behaviours of other healthcare professionals and the patient (Moulton and King 2010), and are powerful in altering the social and moral status of vulnerable older persons. Medicine's codes and conventions, such as strong risk avoidance, and a focus on physical outcomes, can frame the approach in the capacity assessment, thus becoming a form of social control. Medicine's expanding 'gaze' (Foucault 2000: 129) leads to greater scrutiny of persons once they become defined as patients than when they are living in the everyday world. They become subject to detailed observations and examinations, including of cognitive status, and are more vulnerable to direct social control (Waitzkin 1989).

The presence of cognitive frailty in the case study participants was found to diminish the worth of the person and their autonomy. Compliance by the older person was perceived as a sign of insight and capacity, with prejudicial attitudes towards those who were viewed as lacking insight about what would be of benefit to them. The views of family members were often given greater weight than the older person's preferences, and some family members also acquiesced to the healthcare professional's approach to navigating an outcome, relinquishing their own autonomy as well. Such practices exacerbate the loss of social identity and the sense of self in the vulnerable older person, resulting in a weakened ability to resist the imposition of values, and protect one's interests (Benson 2005; Mackenzie and Rogers 2013; Stoljar 2013).

The process of capacity assessment was found to be variable, with common law principles not always evident. Bias by the assessor was evident in two cases, influencing the priorities for decision-making. Assumptions were also made about the older person's cognitive impairment, affecting attitudes and behaviour. Further, an analysis of the assessment and decision-making process by healthcare staff indicated that outcomes were often decided upon by the healthcare team independently of the older person, whose voice was diminished, with a reliance on seeking assent for a decision already made rather than inclusion in the process. Proposed outcomes for the older person did not often acknowledge or explore the benefits of the older person's preferences and limited their participation in decision-making.

All six cases had either a focus of decision-making on issues of care and accommodation, or were related to the appointment or commencement of substitute decision-makers. These issues are indicative of how medical practice has extended beyond its traditional expertise in the body, to aspects of life where subjective meaning, preferences and relationships are a key dynamic. Assessments into the areas of lifestyle decisions 'medicalise' social conditions and lifestyle transitions, and may extend medical authority over social and personal decisions, way beyond a medical knowledge/training base. This suggests that independent assessors or facilitators of decision-making processes may be necessary to protect those vulnerable to prejudice due to labels of cognitive impairment.

The case studies demonstrated that older people with symptoms of cognitive impairment are highly likely to be ignored, marginalised and disempowered in the healthcare setting. The medicalisation of dementia, with its focus on deficits, and the unquestioned assertion of expertise by healthcare staff beyond healthcare treatments, contributes to the diminishment of the autonomy of older people. Within this context, 'capacity assessment' can become a paternalist tool and a form of social control, removing decision-making rights unnecessarily or inappropriately.

Liberal ideals, with their inherent bias towards a certain notion of rationality, are a limited and thus problematic basis for assessing capacity. This, together with improving knowledge about the capacities of those with dementia, points to the need for an alternative approach to the capacity paradigm. This is particularly necessary in healthcare settings, where power imbalances are marked. It requires recognition by doctors and other healthcare professionals that their attitudes and behaviours can have an effect on the older person's sense of self, and can prejudicially influence the information and options that they offer. This requires knowledge about the harm that can result from exclusion of people from decision-making about their lives and imposed solutions to life's challenges by those with greater power.

The intertwined nature of autonomy and personhood was evident from the case studies, where those with physical and mental frailties experienced a reduction in autonomy and personhood, resulting in the imposition of values and constrained choices. The findings suggest that alternative processes are required for navigating and supporting decision-making for those currently considered 'lesser' persons due to the presence of or assumptions about cognitive impairment.

## Seeking a new approach

An alternative approach to that of capacity needs to maximise the autonomy of the older person through recognition of their strengths, respect for their preferences and participation in decision-making. This moves the focus from the expertise and authority of the treating health professionals to their relationship with the patient, requiring openness and empathy. In contrast to the paternalistic approaches that liberalism encourages, where protection justifies intervention, this approach seeks to have both the ends and the means of decision-making enhance autonomy and recognise a wider spectrum of personal capacities.

A broader view of autonomy is to recognise that it is shaped within relationships and by social norms. This leads to the understanding that autonomy is relative to each person in his or her context, rather than an absolute state. Understanding autonomy is central to the sense of self and subsequent well-being, and, therefore, it is essential to enhance an older person's participation in decisions about their lives. With an understanding of autonomy as relational, the goal becomes that of creating the environment, practices and relationships that can maximise autonomy and sense of self, and with it, optimal functioning and wellbeing. A relational approach to autonomy allows a model to be developed for application in medical and service settings that can better support decision-making processes that are respectful of personhood.

An exploration of literature shows a number of alternative approaches to the cognitive rational capacity approach, each with different emphases. These have been grouped to reflect their main approach. The first, which I describe as the *combined substantive/procedural* approach, assesses the person's understanding of the decision, coupled with exploring the subjective meaning for the person (Breden and Vollman 2004). A variation on this approach lies in exploring the different values of the person and others where a conflict about the outcome has led to the assessment, and seeking a negotiated solution where possible, as an alternative to assessment (Darzins *et al.* 2000).

The *partnership* approach recognises the residual autonomy of the person but also that assistance with decision-making may be needed. The approach by Glass (1997) also offers advocacy for the person, while Flynn and Arnstein-Kerslake (2014) maintain that most people with cognitive disabilities can, with the appropriate support, make the decision independently, and where this is not possible, places the person's preferences as central to substitute decision-making, rejecting a 'best interests' approach.

The *presumption of capacity* approach treats the person as competent and with an intact value system that has developed over their lifetime, demonstrated through consistency in choices (Dubler 1985). Within this grouping, Herring (2009) gives status to the person's views and feelings in respect for their right to dignity and liberty, only intervening if serious harm may result.

In the *hermeneutic/narrative* approach, respect is given to the worldview of the person, requiring an understanding of how the person interprets and responds to the world, and modifying the environment to empower the person in their situation (Benaroyo and Widdershoven 2004). Hughes *et al.* (2006: 18) view the person from the narrative of their life story, engaging in empathic understanding to understand their world, aligning with a person-centred approach to decision-making.

While having different emphases, an essential element in the last three approaches is of maximising the autonomy of the person, rather than testing it. In synthesising elements from these models along with findings from the case studies, I have devised a decision-making model to guide health professionals in the process of engaging older vulnerable persons in healthcare settings, where decisions regarding lifestyle or care are required. The facilitator of the process may be a doctor, psychologist or social worker, but one who is able to be independent from conflicts of interest and has a commitment to ensure that the preferences and interests of the patient are paramount. Family members are also engaged in this process, where otherwise they may have relinquished decision-making to the healthcare team, or colluded with them over the solution.

The process gives priority to enabling the person with dementia to make a decision based on full information and options, with time for consideration and discussion with significant others, and without undue pressure or bias. If the person is unable to participate in the process or comprehend the decision to be made, a formalised assessment of capacity can occur, if necessary, to indicate if a substitute decision-maker is required.

Translating changing ideas about persons with cognitive impairment into reality is complex. This is due to general resistance in the healthcare culture to the underpinning ideology about cognition; the well-entrenched biomedical model with the focus on deficits; and practical implementation in the healthcare setting which operates with its own set of codes, conventions and regulations. To this extent, the proposed model is aspirational, promoting an ideal. However, similar practices being incorporated in the disability sector are representative of future possibilities in aged care services for people with dementia (Bigby and Douglas 2015).

## The relational decision-making model

The relational model described below supports the older person with cognitive impairment to participate in the decision-making process, by listening to their expressed preferences and identifying and expanding options that are congruent. It involves family members and incorporates their knowledge and concerns, recognising the significance of these relationships. The relational model also identifies where the imposition of value judgements and conflicts of interest may result in unnecessary restrictions, manipulation or control. The model recognises the need for support in decision-making, aligning with comparative approaches in the emerging area of supporting decision-making in the disability sector, where service providers are encouraged to facilitate the participation of the individual in decision-making about their goals (Bigby and Douglas 2015).

Where significant barriers prevent the resolution of the problem using this relational approach, the legal capacity model, as guided by common law, acts as the default mechanism. The traditional legal capacity approach, as a default, enables essential consent for treatment by healthcare professionals, through the person either having a legal capacity to make the decision, or the substitute decision-maker taking responsibility for the decision. This acknowledges law's function in mediating the problems that arise in human relationships (Kerridge *et al.* 1998; Naffine 2009).

As different laws have different purposes, there may be a perceived tension in the medical setting with interpretations of other aspects of law, which may contradict the relational approach. For instance, duty of care can often be interpreted by health professionals through the lens of risk aversion, and may be used to impose protections on the patient, rather than that of balancing risks and benefits and minimising risks. This form of medical paternalism can be justified by the health professional through reference to the law, and works against the relational approach. In general, greater education about the law in health settings will be of benefit to health professionals in understanding the role of law in everyday practice (White *et al.* 2016).

I propose five main stages of the relational decision-making model, followed by the default position. They are: assuming capacity; knowing the person and their preferences; identifying and creating congruent choices; supporting the person in the decision-making process; and assisting with the plan and its implementation. Where a shared resolution is not obtained, a default capacity approach can indicate if the person is unable to participate meaningfully and substitute decision-making is required. If so, the substitute decision-maker becomes an advocate for the older person, to keep the preferences and life meaning of that person central. The model relies on the development of relationships between health professionals and the older person. I elaborate below, using Andrei's case study to illustrate how this model would have impacted in each stage. It commences at the point that a significant decision is required with no simple negotiated resolution apparent.

## *Assuming capacity*

This stage comprises viewing the older person as capable of participating in decision-making, but recognising that they may need assistance in this process. Respect for the person and their views are paramount. In Andrei's situation, this would have been represented by openness and attention to his will and preferences, and full inclusion in discussions related to his healthcare and future.

## *Knowing the person*

This stage involves an understanding of the older person's history and current life meaning, their strengths and their relationships with significant others. Perspectives of the healthcare team and significant others are gathered by the facilitator, and any conflicts of interests identified. In Andrei's case, this would have translated into identifying his preferences in the current context, recognising his personal strengths that may contribute to the options and those who are significant in relationship to him, along with their values and concerns. Dialogue about these aspects may facilitate the identification of resources and opportunities. In this stage supports for disabilities such as his blindness would be identified and offered.

## *Identifying and creating choices*

In this stage, options are given attention: exploring, identifying, creating and maximising choices for the older person in relation to their situation and preferences. Risks, resources and restraints are identified. In Andrei's situation, attention would be given to supports that would facilitate his choice in living at home, such as meals, hygiene care, social opportunities and resources that would assist him in managing his blindness. Access to these resources and costs are identified, and specific risks and benefits weighed up. Family members are engaged in this process, enabling assumptions and challenges to be explored.

### Supporting decision-making

Assistance for the person in understanding the facts and consequences takes place. Several conversations may be required in order to assist Andrei to comprehend the issues and potential options. There is time to reflect on the concerns of others and possible risks, along with resource issues and dialogue with significant others. Time is spent with Andrei discussing the relevant information, choices and concerns of others, and there is ongoing dialogue with significant others. A decision is reached with support of significant others.

### Establishing and activating the plan

With resolution of the decision, a plan is developed in collaboration with significant others, incorporating the assistance required and access to resources. For Andrei's situation, this involves developing a plan in collaboration with all parties and activating the assistance and resources to enact it.

### The capacity approach as default

If the issue remains unresolved despite assistance, or unsurmountable barriers restrict enacting the person's choice, legal capacity of the person is assessed. This process requires a procedural approach towards decision-making ability, with the goal to ascertain who makes the decision, not what the outcome is. From the capacity assessment, the older person makes the decision if passing the 'understanding' threshold, and if not, the substitute decision-maker takes on this responsibility. In the latter situation, support is given to the substitute decision-maker in making the decision with due regard for the person's preferences within the context and resources, and assisted to develop and enact a plan. In Andrei's situation, the assessor focuses on Andrei's understanding of the different choices and their consequences, not making a judgement on the outcome of the decision. If Andrei was seen as not having capacity to make the decision, his substitute decision-maker would be supported to give primary focus to Andrei's preferences with the resources identified to assist, and to activate the plan.

## Conclusion

This chapter has indicated some of the instances and ways that the legal and social personhood of older persons with cognitive impairment is eroded, personally and socially, through the diminishing of their autonomy. Labels of dementia or cognitive impairment, whether assumed or actual, can lead to prejudicial behaviours such as exclusion and paternalism. These behaviours not only diminish the social status of the person but reduce their sense of self, which in turn effects the expression of that autonomy.

There is a challenge in broadening society's insights about the older person who experiences cognitive disorders. This requires ways of communicating alternative ideas about persons with cognitive changes, and greater awareness of stereotypes and beliefs that influence practice. In the healthcare environment, with its power imbalances, there is an imperative to ensure fair and just approaches by health professionals towards older persons in their care.

The case studies illustrate that greater attention to the harms arising from the limited focus on the deficits of the older person is required, and increased under-standing of the effects of labels and subsequent prejudicial responses. Ignoring power differentials, not listening to the person, and not taking social relation-ships into account, can lead to poor outcomes for older people. The majority of those in the case studies were offered no other choices than residential care, had no choice but to be compliant, and experienced significant loss as a result. The outcomes could have been very different if their wishes were respected and their participation in decision-making supported.

Respecting and enabling the decision-making of older persons is recognised by the Australian Law Reform Commission (2017) as a significant and urgent requirement. The law has a role to facilitate these changes that alter attitudes towards those with cognitive impairment. Additionally, new responses in health-care practices that empower and support the older person in decision-making are necessary. This will necessitate the development of specific principles, policies and processes within each healthcare setting to aid in the implementation of a respectful approach to decision-making. This can be assisted by resources to support the facilitation role in decision-making, the provision of independent capacity assessors where necessary and ongoing education in the healthcare setting.

## Note

1 The concept of capacity for decision-making has its basis in common law doctrines of informed consent. Legal principles applied in tests for legal incompetence are that capacity is presumed; that incapacity is to be proven and related to brain impairment; that capacity is based on the understanding of the decision and not dependent on the outcome; that capacity is decision specific and variable, and that the threshold for capa-city is to be commensurate with the gravity of the decision (see Kerridge *et al.* 2009). These principles can be overridden by specific legislation but otherwise should form the basis of any medical assessment. Most significantly, the test is on the ability to understand the decision and its consequences, and not on whether the outcome is wise – if there is resulting evidence that a person has reached the threshold of understanding, they maintain their freedom to make the decision in this specific matter (see Darzins *et al.* 2000).

## References

Agich, G., 1990, Reassessing autonomy in long-term care, *The Hastings Center Report*, 20(6): 12–17.

Alzheimer's Australia, 2011, *Pfizer Health Report Dementia: Dementia is Everyone's Business*, https://fight dementia.org.au/research-and-publications/reports-and-publications/pfizer-health-reports [Accessed 18 June 2014].

Alzheimer's Australia, 2014, *Living with Dementia Program*, https://fightdementia.org.
au/sites/default/files/20140612_-_National_-_Services_Support_-_Living_with_
Dementia.pdf [Accessed 30 March 2015].

Alzheimer's Australia, 2017, *Statistics*, www.fightdementia.org.au/statistics [Accessed 21
June 2017].

Australian Law Reform Commission., 2017, *Elder Abuse: A National Legal Response*,
Summary Report 131, www.alrc.gov.au/sites/default/files/pdfs/publications/31_may_
summary_report_131_0.pdf [Accessed 27 June 2017].

Batsch, N., M. Mittelman, 2012, *World Alzheimer Report 2012: Overcoming the Stigma
of Dementia*, London: Alzheimer's Disease International, www.alz.org/documents_
custom/ world_report_2012_final.pdf [Accessed 21 February 2014].

Behuniak, S., 2011, The living dead? The construction of people with Alzheimer's
disease as zombies, *Ageing and Society*, 31: 70–92.

Benaroyo, L., G. Widdershoven, 2004, Competence in mental health care: A hermeneutic
perspective, *Health Care Analysis*, 12: 295–298.

Benson, P., 1994, Free agency and self-worth, *Journal of Philosophy*, 91: 650–668.

Benson, P., 2005, Feminist intuitions and the normative substance of autonomy, in J.S.
Taylor (ed.), *Personal Autonomy: New Essays on Personal Autonomy and its Role in
Contemporary Moral Philosophy*, pp. 124–142, Cambridge, UK: Cambridge Univer-
sity Press.

Bigby, C., J. Douglas, 2015, *Support for Decision Making: A Practice Framework*, Australia: Living with Disability Research Centre, La Trobe University.

Bigby, C., M. Whiteside, J. Douglas, 2015, *Supporting People with Cognitive Disabilities
in Decision Making: Processes and Dilemmas*, Melbourne, Australia: Living with
Disability Research Centre, La Trobe University.

Bond, J., 1992, The medicalization of dementia, *Journal of Ageing Studies*, 6(4):
397–403.

Bond, J., L. Corner, A. Lilley, C. Ellwood, 2002, Medicalization of insight and caregivers' responses to risk in dementia, *Dementia*, 1(3): 313–328.

Breden, T.M., J. Vollman, 2004, The cognitive based approach of capacity assessment in
psychiatry: A philosophical critique of the MacCAT-T, *Health Care Analysis*, 273: 276.

Bredesen, D., 2014, Reversal of cognitive decline: A novel therapeutic program, *Aging*,
6(9): 707–717.

Brooker, D., 2004, What is person-centred care in dementia?, *Reviews in Clinical Gerontology*, 13: 215–222.

Brown, I., R. Brown, 2009, Choice as an aspect of quality of life for people with intellectual disability, *Journal of Policy and Practice in Intellectual Disabilities*, 6(1): 11–18.

Bryden, C., 2012, *Who Shall I Be When I Die?*, London: Jessica Kingsley Publishers.

Carney, T., 1991, *Law at the Margins*, Melbourne, Australia: Oxford University Press.

Charland, L., 1998, Is Mr Spock mentally competent: Competence to consent and
emotion, *Philosophy, Psychiatry, Psychology*, 5(1): 67–81.

Christman, J., 2003, Autonomy in moral and political philosophy, *The Stanford Encyclo-
paedia of Philosophy*, http://plato.stanford.edu/entries/autonomy-moral/ [Accessed 11
December 2008].

Clarke, C., H. Wilkinson, J. Keady, D. Gibb, 2011, *Risk Assessment and Management for
Living Well with Dementia*, London: Jessica Kingsley Publishers.

Cuddy, A., S. Fiske, 2004, Doddering but dear: Process, content, and function in stereotyping of older persons, in T. Nelson (ed.), *Ageism: Stereotyping and Prejudice Against
Older Persons*, pp. 3–26, Paperback edition, Massachusetts, USA: MIT Press.

Darzins, P., D.W. Molloy, D. Strang, 2000, *Who Can Decide? The Six Step Capacity Assessment Process*, Adelaide, Australia: Memory Australia Press.

Davis, D., 2004, Dementia: Sociological and philosophical constructions, *Social Science and Medicine*, 28: 369–378.

Deci, E., 1980, *The Psychology of Self-Determination*, Maryland, USA: Lexington Books.

Devereaux, J., M. Parker, 2006, Competency issues for young persons and older persons, in I. Freckleton and K. Peterson (eds), *Disputes and Dilemmas in Healthcare*, pp. 54–76, Sydney: The Federation Press.

Dubler, N.N., 1985, Some legal and moral issues surrounding informed consent for treatment and research involving the cognitively impaired elderly, in M.B. Kapp, H.E. Pies, A.E. Doudera (eds), *Legal and Ethical Aspects of Health Care*, pp. 247–257, Ann Arbor, USA: Health Administration Press.

Dworkin, G., 1971, Paternalism, in R. Wasserstrom (ed.), *Morality and the Law*, pp. 107–126, Belmont, USA: Wadsworth.

Epp, T.D., 2003, Person-centred dementia care: A vision to be refined, *The Canadian Alzheimer Disease Review*, April.

Faden, R., T. Beauchamp, N. King, 1986, *History and Theory of Informed Consent*, New York: Oxford University Press.

Flynn, E., A. Arstein-Kerslake, 2014, Legislating personhood: Realising the right to support in exercising legal capacity, *International Journal of Law in Context*, 10(1): 81–104.

Foucault, M., 2000, *The Birth of the Clinic: An Archaeology of Medical Perception*, London: Routledge.

Glass, K., 1997, Redefining definitions and devising instruments: Two decades of assessing competence, *International Journal of Law and Psychiatry*, 20: 1–29.

Goffman, E., 1961, *Asylums: Essays on the Social Situation of Mental Patients and Other Inmates*, Garden City, USA: Anchor Books.

Herring, J., 2009, Losing it? Losing what? The law and dementia, *Child and Family Law Quarterly*, 21: 3–26.

Hughes, J.C., S.J. Louw, S. Sabat (eds), 2006, *Dementia: Mind, Meaning and Person*, Oxford, UK: Oxford University Press.

Jaworska, A., 1999, Respecting the margins of agency: Alzheimer's patients and the capacity of value, *Philosophy and Public Affairs*, 28(2): 105–138.

Kerridge, I., M. Lowe, S. McPhee, 1998, *Ethics and Law for the Health Professions*, Sydney: The Federation Press.

Kerridge, I., M. Lowe, M. Stewart, 2009, *Ethics and Law for the Health Professions*, Sydney, The Federation Press.

Kester, E., 2009, Charles Bonnet syndrome: Case presentation and literature review, *Optometry*, 80(7): 360–366.

Kite, M., L. Wagner, 2004, Attitude towards older adults, in T. Nelson (ed.), *Ageism: Stereotyping and Prejudice Against Older Adults*, Massachusetts, USA: MIT Press.

Kitwood, T., 1997, *Dementia Reconsidered: The Person Comes First*, Buckingham, UK: Open University Press.

Kitwood, T., S. Benson, 1995, *The New Culture of Dementia Care*, London: Hawker.

Kleinig, J., 1983, *Paternalism*, Manchester, UK: Manchester University Press.

Kukathas, C., 1993, Liberty, in R. Goodin and P. Pettit (eds), *A Companion to Contemporary Political Philosophy*, New Jersey, USA: Blackwell.

Lothian, K., I. Philp, 2001, Care of older people: Maintaining the dignity and autonomy of older people in the healthcare setting, *British Medical Journal*, 322(7287): 668–670.

Loveday, B., 2013, *Leadership for Person-Centred Care*, London: Jessica Kingsley Publishers.

Lyman, K., 1989, Bringing the social back in: A critique of the biomedicalization of dementia, *The Gerontologist*, 29(5): 597–605.

Macdonald, G., 2018, Death in life or life in death?: Dementia's ontological challenge, *Death Studies*, 42(5): 290–297.

Mackenzie, C., W. Rogers, 2013, Autonomy, vulnerability and capacity: A philosophical appraisal of the Mental Capacity Act, *International Journal of Law in Context*, 9(1): 37–52.

Maguire, C., M. Kirby, R. Coen, D. Coakley, B. Lawlor, D. O'Neill, 1996, Family members' attitudes toward telling the patient with Alzheimer's disease their diagnosis, *BMJ*, 313(7056): 529–530.

McLeod, C., 2002, *Self-Trust and Reproductive Autonomy*, Cambridge, USA: MIT Press.

Minichiello, V., J. Browne, H. Kendig, 2000, Perceptions and consequences of ageism: Views of older people', *Ageing and Society*, 20(3): 253–278.

Mill, J.S., 1906, *On Liberty*, New York: Alfred A Knopf.

Moulton, B., J. King, 2010, Aligning ethics with medical decision-making: The quest for informed patient choice, *Journal of Law, Medicine and Ethics*, 38(1): 85–97.

Naffine, N., 2009, *Law's Meaning of Life: Philosophy, Religion, Darwin and the Legal Person*, Legal Theory Today, Oxford, UK and Portland, USA: Hart Publishing.

Nay, R., M. Bird, D. Evardsson, R. Fleming, R. Hill, 2009, Person-centred care, in R. Nay, S. Garratt (eds), *Older People: Issues and Innovations in Care*, pp. 137–146, Sydney: Churchill Livingstone, Elsevier.

Nedelsky, J., 2011, *Law's Relations: A Relational Theory of Self, Autonomy, and Law*, New York: Oxford University Press.

Nelson, T., 2005, Ageism: Prejudice against our feared future self, *Journal of Social Issues*, 61(2): 207–221.

O'Connor, D., B. Purves (eds), 2009, *Decision-making, Personhood and Dementia: Exploring the Interface*, London and Philadelphia, USA: Jessica Kingsley Publishers.

Phillipson, L., C. Magee, S. Jones, E. Skladzien, 2012, *Exploring Dementia and Stigma Beliefs*, Canberra, Australia: Alzheimer's Australia.

Post, S., 1995, *The Moral Challenge of Alzheimer's Disease*, Baltimore, USA: The John Hopkins University Press.

Post, S., 2006, Respectare: Moral respect for the lives of the deeply respectful, in J.C. Hughes, S.J. Louw, S. Sabat (eds), *Mind, Meaning, and the Person*, pp. 223–234, Oxford, UK: Oxford University Press.

Power, A., 2014, *Dementia Beyond Disease: Enhancing Well-Being*, Baltimore, USA: Health Professions Press.

Rawls, J., 1971, *A Theory of Justice*, Revised edition (1999), Cambridge, USA: Harvard University Press.

Resnick, L., M. Cowart, A. Kubrin, 1998, Perceptions of do-not-resuscitate orders, *Social Work in Health Care*, 26(4): 1–21.

Stoljar, N., 2013, *Feminist Perspectives on Autonomy*, Stanford, USA: Stanford University, http://plato.stanford.edu/ entries/ feminism-autonomy [Accessed 20 February 2014].

Stone, D., 1991, Caring work in a liberal polity, *Journal of Health Politics, Policy and Law*, 16(3): 547–552.

Surtees, D., 2014, Discrimination, in C. Foster, J. Herring, I. Doron (eds), *The Law and Ethics of Dementia*, pp. 445–455, Oxford, UK: Hart Publishing.

Swaffer, K., 2014, *I Repeat Please Don't Call Us Sufferers*, 11 June, Adelaide, Australia, shttp://kateswaffer.com/2014/05/09/i-repeat-please-don't-call-us-sufferer [Accessed 07 February 2018].

Taylor, R., 2007, *Dementia From the Inside Out*, Baltimore, USA: Health Promotions Press.

Tyrrell, J., N. Genin, M. Myslinski, 2006, Freedom of choice and decision-making in health and social care: Views of older patients with early-stage dementia and their carers, *Dementia*, 5(4): 479–502.

United Nations., 2006, *Convention on the Rights of Persons with Disabilities*, Geneva, Switzerland: UN, www.un.org/disabilities/ convention/ conventionfull.shtml [Accessed 13 May 2015].

Waitzkin, H., 1989, A critical theory of medical discourse: Ideology, social control, and the processing of social context in medical encounters, *Journal of Health and Social Behaviour*, 30: 220–239.

White, B., L., Willmott, C. Cartwright, M. Parker, G. Williams, 2016, The knowledge and practice of doctors in relation to the law that governs withholding and withdrawing life-sustaining treatment from adults who lack capacity, *Journal of Law and Medicine,* 24: 356.

Winick, B., 1996, The side effects of incompetency labelling and the implications for mental health law, in D. Wexler, B. Winick (eds), *Law in a Therapeutic Key: Developments in Therapeutic Jurisprudence*, pp. 17–58, Durham, USA: Carolina Academic Press.

Wood, S., B.E. Tanius, 2007, Impact of dementia on decision-making abilities, in S. Qualls, M. Smyer (eds), *Changes in Decision-Making Capacity in Older Adults: Assessment and Intervention*, Hoboken, USA: John Wiley and Sons.

Woods, B., R. Pratt, 2005, Awareness in dementia: Ethical and legal issues in relation to people with dementia, *Ageing and Mental Health*, 9(5): 423–429.

Woolhead, G., M. Calnan, P. Dieppe, W. Tadd, 2004, Dignity in older age: What do older people in the United Kingdom think?, *Age and Ageing*, 33: 165–170.

# 7 'We've always thought of one another'

## Relational perspectives on autonomy and decision-making among people with dementia and their family carers

*Craig Sinclair, Romola S. Bucks, Meredith Blake, Kathy Williams, Josephine Clayton, Kirsten Auret, Helen Radoslovich, Sascha Callaghan, Sue Field and Susan Kurrle*

### Introduction

Dementia research has demonstrated gradual and progressive changes in brain functions, including language, memory, sensory perception and cognition (Australian Institute of Health and Welfare 2012). Complementing this research on brain functions is a growing body of research focusing on the psychosocial and relational processes associated with dementia. From the early 1990s, Kitwood's theory of dementia care has focused attention on the influence of these processes on the relative wellbeing or ill-being, and enduring 'personhood' of a person with dementia (Kitwood and Bredin 1992; Kitwood 1993, 1997). The cognitive impairments associated with dementia pose challenges in regard to carrying out a range of functional and inter-personal tasks, including decision-making (Samsi and Manthorpe 2013). In the context of decision-making, this shift in thinking has led to revised approaches to understanding the experiences, values and rights of people with dementia, and the importance of maintaining involvement in decision-making about their own lives (O'Connor 2009).

This chapter begins by outlining existing research relating to decision-making in the context of dementia and situating this within broader moral and ethical discourses on the concept of autonomy. In response to this existing literature, and a small number of case studies involving people with dementia and their family carers, we propose that the unique characteristics of the dementia syndrome, and its associated social contexts, can be understood as a stressor at a number of levels (psychosocial, relational and existential). Our work specifically identifies the essential experience of 'stress within relationships' associated with navigating decision-making and applies relational approaches to stress and coping as a way of explaining these experiences.

## Autonomy and decision-making

Inherent in any discussion of decision-making is a consideration of the person or people who are the decision-maker(s) and how they go about this process. Decision-making is often described with reference to the concept of autonomy, which derives from the Greek *auto* ('self') and *nomos* ('rule'), meaning 'self-rule' (Martin *et al.* 2014). The 'autonomous individual', has been described as someone who processes information rationally and exerts agency, acting to shape his or her world and experiences (Series 2015). From this view, decisions are a means by which individuals may pursue their preferred choices with reference to their personal identity, values and goals, and without interference from others. This image of the autonomous individual, 'directing the choir' through the course of their life, is pervasive in western liberal democracies, in which autonomy is privileged (Gysels *et al.* 2012). Such individual agency is encouraged, and often assumed, within contemporary neoliberal discourses of social and healthcare policy, shaping our understanding of decision-making as an individual act.

While the notion of the autonomous individual has dominated ethical and policy discourses on decision-making, there is growing recognition that decision-making is not as rational, or independent, as has been assumed (Gooding 2013). An emerging body of scholarship challenges individualist approaches to autonomy, identifying how social relationships provide the guidance and environment within which people develop and express their capacity for autonomous decision-making (Mackenzie 2008). Others identify how individuals depend on relationships to meaningfully enact decisions (Silvers and Francis 2009). The concept of 'relational autonomy' describes a range of more specific theories, each of which broadly highlight how social relationships and contexts can facilitate or suppress autonomous decision-making. Mackenzie has argued that core attitudes to self, which underpin a person's consideration of themselves as 'able and authorised' to make decisions, are formed through histories of communication and mutual recognition within close relationships (Mackenzie 2008).

At a basic level, supportive or oppressive contexts might facilitate or hinder a person's ability to think through a decision and express a preference. Alternatively, a person's decision might be understood with reference to values shared with important others (e.g. peers or family members) or the primacy of maintaining valued relationships, or relational roles (e.g. the 'devoted daughter', or the 'good provider') over other considerations. Finally, the relational approach also sensitises us to sources of inequality and undue influence which can exist within relationships, and their impact on decision-making (Ho 2008). These can be the product of structural factors in society (e.g. age or gender inequality) which are further exacerbated in the context of vulnerability associated with dementia.

The concept of relational autonomy thus provides an alternative perspective for interpreting a person's decision, as well as informing ethical arguments on the related obligations of others to respect these decisions. In the context of dementia, these obligations may extend to promoting the relational and contextual conditions within which people with dementia can most readily enjoy and express their autonomy.

## Dementia and decision-making

People with dementia have identified the importance of remaining in control of decisions about their lifestyle and care (Fetherstonhaugh *et al.* 2013). However, the progressive nature of the cognitive impairments associated with dementia means that some people, in some situations, will lack the necessary decision-making capacity to understand and weigh the consequences of the decision at hand, or to communicate their preferences (Gregory *et al.* 2007). In these situations, the conventional approach has been to turn to substitute decision-makers (often close family members), who apply a 'substituted judgment' ('stepping into the person's shoes' to make the decision they would have made) or 'best interest' approach (Hirschman *et al.* 2006).

However, Rhoden (1990) has argued persuasively that the nature of incapacity for those with age-related impairments, who have had the chance to form values over a 'life long-lived' is substantively different to those who have never been able to make decisions. Research has shown difficulties associated with substitute decision-making in this context, including discrepancies between the ratings of values and preferences by people with dementia, compared with family caregivers (Reamy *et al.* 2011). Those assuming responsibilities as substitute decision-makers for people with dementia also describe a range of practical, inter-personal, moral and financial challenges on what has been described as a 'difficult and unpredictable journey' (Fetherstonhaugh *et al.* 2017: 22).

Given these challenges, significant effort has been invested in encouraging members of the public, including people diagnosed with dementia, to 'plan ahead' for future decisions (Australian Health Minister's Advisory Council 2011; Cognitive Decline Partnership Centre 2016). Planning ahead can be seen as a form of anticipatory decision-making, covering a range of issues (e.g. lifestyle, accommodation, healthcare, financial and estate) and an extended time-period (short-term, long-term and post-death). However, people with dementia and their family members have identified challenges associated with planning ahead, including uncertain symptom burden and prognosis (Dickinson *et al.* 2013), lack of information and support from health professionals (Brown and Jarrad 2008) and difficulty in discussing end-of-life issues (Hirschman *et al.* 2008).

We propose that challenges associated with decision-making in the context of dementia can be understood in relation to the known and feared trajectory of cognitive, physical and *social* losses for people diagnosed with the condition (Brannelly 2011), along with the associated impacts on family members, relationships and broader social networks. We therefore understand the need for decision-making associated with dementia as a stressor, and peoples' responses as a form of coping.

## Individual and relational theories of coping

The 1980s saw the development of influential theories relating to how people interpret and cope with stressors associated with chronic illness. Charmaz (1983) described how chronic illness challenges one's 'sense of self', through loss of identities, loss of roles and ongoing existential threat. Lazarus and Folkman (1984) developed a transactional model in which individuals appraise situations or events, identifying the demands placed on them, and the resources available to cope with these demands. Where the demands of coping with the threat outweigh available resources, stress would result. Based on this appraisal, individuals invoke coping strategies that can broadly be categorised as problem-focused (aimed at fixing the problem) or emotion-focused (aimed at reducing negative emotions associated with the stressor).

More recently, Berg and colleagues have described a number of dyadic models of coping with chronic illness, which are attuned to the relational way in which illness-related stressors may be *interdependently* (as opposed to independently) appraised (Berg *et al.* 1998; Berg and Upchurch 2007). The type of stressor appraisal influences the ways that people tend to relate to one another in coping with the stressor (see Table 7.1). These *coping configurations* can be broadly seen on a spectrum of relational interactions, ranging from uninvolvement, through to support, collaboration and control (Berg *et al.* 1998). Interdependent stressor appraisal (seeing the problem as 'ours') is associated with the engagement of supportive and collaborative coping configurations, and has been associated with better adjustment and outcomes (Häusler *et al.* 2016).

Factors associated with adopting interdependent appraisals and coping strategies in response to illness-related stressors include female gender, 'collectivist'

*Table 7.1* Dyadic configurations for stressor appraisal (adapted from Berg *et al.*, 1998)

| Configuration | Level of interdependence | Description |
| --- | --- | --- |
| Solitary individual | Low | An individual appraises the problem on their own, and sees it as their problem |
| Parallel individual | Moderate | Two individuals in a given context perceive the problem differently, or bring different individual characteristics to the problem, leading to different appraisals and coping responses |
| Indirect relational | Moderate | One individual of a dyad appraises a problem as stressful, this stress affects the other person indirectly, but not to the extent that the other person defines the problem as their own |
| Shared relational | High | Both individuals appraise the problem as stressful, and shared with the other member of the dyad. The stressor cannot be characterised as belonging to just one or other individual |

(as opposed to individualist) cultural background, relationship factors (e.g. marital quality) and illness-related factors (time course, daily management needs, impacts on cognition and communication abilities, impacts on relationships, ability to exert control, impacts on identity).

## Experiences of decision-making

The remainder of this chapter asks whether Berg and collaborators' dyadic coping theory can provide a useful way of operationalising the relational contexts in which decision-making is experienced by people with dementia and their family members. We draw on four in-depth interviews with six people in different relational and gender configurations in which participants explore decision-making relating to admission to residential care. Two of the interviews were individual and two were with dyads (one husband-wife, one parent-child), highlighting the social and relational aspects of the decision-making experience (Samsi and Manthorpe 2013). Due to the impacts of dementia on roles, identity and relationships, we conceptualise the 'need' for decisions triggered by dementia as a stressor, and collaborative engagement with decision-making as one form of coping. This small-scale study is not intended to support a comprehensive conclusion about the lived experiences of decision-making by people with dementia, but instead to demonstrate the utility of a relational perspective in understanding how people respond to the stressors associated with decision-making.

We employed a 'process consent' approach to obtaining (and maintaining) informed consent (Dewing 2007). Partnerships with aged care service providers and Alzheimer's Australia enabled identification of eligible people with dementia (formally diagnosed and assessed by service providers as 'mild to moderate' severity) and family carers. Senior staff (such as facility care managers, programme coordinators) facilitated introductions to the researcher, who met informally with potential participants to build rapport and explain the study.

The interviewer (CS) used a semi-structured discussion guide, which focused on participants' previous experiences of decision-making (including examples), typical approaches to decision-making and thoughts about decision-making in the future. The interviews were digitally recorded, transcribed verbatim and analysed using an Interpretative Phenomenological Analysis approach (Smith *et al.* 2009), with the concepts of relational autonomy and dyadic coping theory as guiding theoretical perspectives (Berg and Upchurch 2007; Mackenzie 2008; Epstein 2013). In each case, we considered how participants described relationships and how this helped explain their reflections on decision-making. The study was approved by the University of Western Australia Human Research Ethics Committee (RA/4/1/8307) and pseudonyms are used to protect participant identities.

### Josie (person with dementia, age 75 years)

Josie is a retired nurse who lives at home with her husband in a regional area. She reported experiencing cognitive changes five years prior to the interview, and was formally diagnosed with dementia two years later. She described her experience of the impact of dementia on her sense of self-confidence in undertaking tasks, making everyday decisions and going on social outings. Fluctuating symptoms meant that some days she would feel capable of making decisions, while other days she would 'just freeze'. Her difficulties in making decisions were a challenge to her self-identity and role within her marital relationship: 'I've always been the decision-maker. I've always been the one that's done the banking'. While her husband attempted to help Josie maintain involvement (through writing monthly financial statements in a book, so that she could monitor expenses), this was only sometimes effective. In addition to her own emotional experience post-diagnosis 'I think I cried for three months and then I got angry', Josie spoke about difficulties communicating with her husband, and his difficulty understanding her experience. These relationship factors impacted on her self-confidence and ability to cope:

> I have no confidence anymore, it's gone ... Probably because I feel as though I've been battened [sic] down a lot by my husband. But it's not his fault, don't get me wrong, I'm not blaming him. But because he couldn't understand, it's been an awful thing for him. So it's been a constant shouting match at times because I've never been one to sit back and let people walk all over me.

In talking about future decisions, Josie was clear about her wishes, which included discussions with her husband about future living arrangements:

> I made the decision to go in a home [residential aged care facility], which [husband] was dead against ... Well, right from the word go [husband] said 'No. We've married for better for worse. I will look after you.' I said 'you won't cope.' So he said 'yes I will, yes I will, I'll learn to cope.'... He realizes now he will not cope.

While this presents initially as an example of Josie making and advocating for her own decision, her reflections on the process explain it as an example of how she and her husband had considered one another:

> [Husband]'s in agreement with me now. Which is good ... But he didn't like it at first, but I had to – we've always thought of one another. It's going to be hard for him anyway, whichever way it goes... but it will be a lot easier for him if I'm in a home [residential aged care facility]... I love him too much to put that sort of thing onto him.

Josie's reflections on decision-making, 'it will be a lot easier for him', illustrate her relational frame of reference in her decision-making about future living arrangements, which reflected their historical approach 'we've always thought of one another'. Her description aligns with Berg *et al.*'s (1998) description of a 'parallel individual' coping configuration, in which they initially understand the challenge of coping with dementia from different perspectives. Josie's husband refers to his personal commitment to the 'marital contract', reflecting an individualist approach which sees his care for Josie as a 'one-way' commitment: 'I will learn to cope'. Josie takes a broader view which considers the wellbeing of both partners and the quality of the relationship. Based on her narrative, it could be argued that their approach transitions towards a more mutual acceptance around future living arrangements, aligning with the 'shared relational' configuration. However, without the direct perspective of Josie's husband, it is difficult to know whether his acceptance reflects a change in his perspective (greater consideration of both partners' needs and their mutual impacts on the relationship) or simply a realisation that 'he will not cope' within an ongoing individualist framework.

### Judy (carer, age 68 years)

Judy is a carer for her husband, who was diagnosed with vascular dementia subsequent to a stroke (which occurred 12 years before interview). They live together in a suburban home with their daughter, who works full-time, and Judy receives regular assistance from a day respite service. Judy spoke about her experience of progressively taking on more of the decision-making and household tasks, including those 'which I call men things':

> To begin with, he'd say 'I can't think, I can't sort that out, I don't know'. Then it's graduated so that he's sort of accepted that I'm the one making the decisions – he's just drifted into it if you like, and I guess so have I.

Judy described a sense of discomfort and burden associated with the more independent approach to decision-making:

> I felt the burden of not having someone to share the responsibility. We always talked about stuff. We've been married a long time and it was all our money, not one or the other and we made decisions about money between us ... I don't know quite what I felt but I didn't like doing it on my own. Like I say, now I've gotten used to it but that was a big thing.

As her husband's condition deteriorated further his care needs increased to the point where he needed to be discharged by one of his day care providers, leaving Judy contemplating the difficult decision of having her husband admitted to residential aged care:

> I really at that stage wasn't ready for him to go into aged care on a permanent basis. I don't know if I am ready still but I am because I need to be

because I can't cope. Emotionally I feel bad about it. I don't want it to happen but it's got to happen ...

Part of this emotional conflict was related to her husband's growing need to be with Judy constantly, and her need to reassure him, despite her private thoughts about this looming decision:

whether he's got some inkling that he might be going somewhere else, I don't know but he's been very, very... the last three or four months is very 'I want you, I'm with you.' And I mean, I try to reassure him. We don't actually usually tell lies, even white ones to each other but I do. I say, 'No [husband], I'm always going to be. I'm here. We're always going to be together.' What else can I say?

Judy's reflections on decision-making illustrate her sense of loss and discomfort associated with feeling forced into a more independent approach to decision-making, which aligns with Berg *et al.*'s (1998) description of a 'solitary individual' coping configuration. She is further constrained by a lack of suitable options that might enable her husband's increasing care needs to be managed, while staying at home. She describes how these factors position her in a carer role in relation to her husband, trying to 'cope' and 'reassure', compared with the more open and mutual spousal relationship she previously had. She also observes how the decision about residential care admission will impact them both.

### Derek (person with dementia, age 71 years) and June (carer, age 67 years)

Derek is a retired engineer, who was diagnosed with dementia five years prior to the interview, shortly after relocating to a regional city with his wife June. A recent fall and hip fracture had triggered his move into residential care, which they were both already planning for him. June described how she interpreted the diagnosis of dementia as a problem for both of them: 'you sort of think, why us? Why is it happening to us'? The stress of this news, and the decisions they made in response, were processed in the context of a strong and open relationship: 'I think we're lucky that we've been able to talk things through together – it's been good. I don't envy those trapped couples that have the difficulty of decisions and denial with what's going on' (June).

Derek described the importance of accepting help and advice. This was described as a process of transition 'it was a bit hard to do that at first', but was described in relation to his pragmatic approach to coping:

I've always been fairly pragmatic about things. If a big heavy thing is coming out of the sky is going to fall on your head, there's nothing you can do about it – you know what I mean – and so you learn to avoid it or accept it.

Both endorsed this open and 'pragmatic' approach, which focused on 'just get[ting] on and talking about it'. They went to their financial adviser and 'told him completely' about the dementia diagnosis and their need to make changes to Derek's superannuation. June would attend Derek's appointments 'I'd listen and put my bit in ... and I'd take note of all the information' and Derek felt supported by her 'just being there... it gives you confidence'. Derek described a positive experience of completing an advance care directive in relation to his future medical treatment 'it's a weight off your shoulder [*sic*]'.

In spite of their open approach, June also reflected on how the illness had led to increased tension in their relationship, 'mainly because I'd get tired and... uptight and stressed and you [kept] pushing, pushing'. This had contributed to their decision to seek a residential care placement for Derek. June felt this had had a positive impact on their relationship, 'I'm much more tolerant [now]', and Derek, while unable to recall this period of their relationship, reflected on how the shift to residential care '...was a very good idea... it takes a bit of a weight off June'.

Derek and June's interdependent stressor appraisal (identifying problems as 'ours') and sharing a similar perspective of taking an open approach to discussion and decision-making, in which both consider each other's needs, aligns with Berg *et al.*'s (1998) conception of a 'shared relational' coping approach. Both described this approach as contributing to their ability to move through an initial stage of emotion-focused coping, towards a joint, problem-focused approach to decision-making.

### Ruth (person with dementia, age 79 years) and Steven (carer, age 46 years)

Ruth is an older lady, who until the recent death of her husband was living in her home in a regional town. Her fear of living on her own far away from other family, and concerns from her children, had prompted a move to the city, to live with her son Steven and his family in their home. However, this situation soon became difficult for Steven's family, leading to his decision to move Ruth into a nearby residential care facility. Steven participated in the interview with Ruth, and described how his father's death had revealed Ruth's difficulties managing at home on her own, which had triggered himself and his brother into becoming more involved in Ruth's care: 'As soon as Dad died, that was it, the shit hit the fan and we had to find out what was going on. And we didn't know the progression [of the dementia] back then to what we know now'.

Steven had initiated an Enduring Power of Attorney for himself and his brother, 'that's what I had Mum do just before', so that they could make arrangements for Ruth's care and the sale of her house. He described his perception of being responsible for key decisions about Ruth's health care '...the decision for taking the gall bladder out was my decision', and rationalised this using a 'best interest' approach which privileged Ruth's physical safety and balanced the risks of the operation against the risks of future infection, '...so it was better off taking it out', without reference to her wishes. He found the aged care system complex and financial decision-making confusing:

> So I'm blindfolded to what goes on. I mean we're in the dark, the same as anything that happens. You never go through it, so you're always in the dark when it happens. And there's not many resources out there to point you along the way.

Ruth described her general satisfaction with her children making decisions for her 'I'll leave it to the pair of them... as long as they do what I would like them to be doing'. She perceived that they would implicitly understand her wishes, on the basis that 'they pretty well knew me', a view which Steven endorsed: '...we've never talked about any of these sort of things but, like she said, we know Mum so we know what she wants'. However, he also noted constraints on enacting these wishes: 'Just sometimes we can't give her what she wants. Like sometimes we have to sacrifice'.

While Ruth endorsed Steven's acknowledgement of the constraints he faced in making decisions for her, both she and Steven also contested some decisions, while others were not acknowledged. Steven confided after the interview that he saw Ruth's move into residential care as an unfortunate necessity, as he and his family were unable to cope with caring for her at home, along with their work commitments. He stated that Ruth 'thinks she's in a church camp'. Ruth's responses during the interview were consistent with this, but also suggested her wishes to avoid residential care:

> RUTH: 'I'm not going into a home, that's for sure'
> STEVEN: 'No we wouldn't do that Mum'
> RUTH: 'Yeah you keep telling me that love'

It is notable that, while Steven contested a number of Ruth's claims in the interview on the basis of her memory loss (for example, whether she had access to a phone and agreements about when he would visit), Ruth's perception about being in a church camp was not challenged. It could be that this reflected Steven's strategy of not challenging Ruth's belief, and that this omission functioned to protect both of them from the more confronting relational impacts that might occur if they openly discussed Ruth's placement in residential care, which was against her expressed wishes. While this approach is disempowering for Ruth in terms of her lack of access to information, it may be that in the absence of meaningful alternatives, such an omission is intended to spare Ruth from distress associated with her wishes being overridden, or Steven's own concerns about her reactions towards him. In this way, their avoidance of open discussion about this decision could be seen as a type of emotion-focused coping, deriving from a parallel relational coping configuration (Berg *et al.* 1998), in which the two members of the dyad perceive the problem differently, and require some means of integrating their conflicting views, while maintaining a valued relationship.

It is of course notable that Steven is placed in a position of power in the relationship, having the choice to remind Ruth about the reality of her living arrangement.

## Implications

In describing their experiences, participants foregrounded a number of issues that justify understanding decision-making in the context of dementia as a stressor. These include the challenges of the illness, to identity, roles and relationships, as well as the nature of the decisions required, many of which were complex, unanticipated and time-pressured, with implications for peoples' ongoing relationships. In the context of clinical decision-making, Epstein has argued that it is these contexts in which a relational perspective on decision-making is particularly important (Epstein 2013). We now explore the extent to which these participant experiences can be usefully interpreted from a relational perspective, by discussing the data with reference to Berg *et al.*'s (1998) developmental-contextual model of dyadic coping.

In common with other dyadic coping theories, Berg *et al.*'s (1998) model proposes that stressors are jointly appraised by both members of the dyad, who each enact coping responses in ways which mutually interact, influencing both members and their ongoing relationship. These coping responses are formed with reference to developmental histories in the relationship, as well as the current context in which the stressor is appraised. Based on this appraisal and individual coping responses, the theory proposes that the *dyadic* response can be characterised by one of their dyadic coping configurations (shared relational, parallel individual, indirect relational and solitary individual). A substantial body of research on coping with chronic illness has suggested that interdependent stressor appraisals (seeing the problem as 'ours') and a shared relational coping configuration, is associated with more adaptive coping responses (Berg and Upchurch 2007). It is important to note, however, that the majority of this research has been conducted in the context of heterosexual spouse couples. Although application of dyadic coping theory in dementia research is still in its early stages, one recent study has shown that 'dyadic coping', as measured by a validated questionnaire, mediates the relationship between self-reported stress and quality of life for carers of people with dementia (Häusler *et al.* 2016). This suggests the relevance of exploring the utility of this theory in understanding the stressors associated with decision-making in the context of a diagnosis of dementia.

In line with dyadic coping theories, our case studies suggest that decision-making stressors were appraised by both members of the dyad – in respect of themselves and the other person. Interdependent stressor appraisal, and explicit identification of problems as 'ours', as in the example of Derek and June, was explained with reference to the strength of the relationship, and a history of making decisions together. They linked this approach with the use of more supportive and collaborative styles of coping and decision-making.

However, even for people who reported a history of interdependent stressor appraisal and collaborative decision-making, the progression of dementia introduced challenges to their preferred approach. For Judy, changes in her habitual approaches to joint decision-making with her husband, along with the broader loss of mutuality in their relationship and enforcement of a 'carer role' with the progression of dementia, were described as challenging. For Josie, she attributed a change in her husband's willingness to accept her consideration for his well-being in addition to her own, with reference to his gradual acceptance of her dementia. Such observations are consistent with existing literature, and suggest that coping configurations can change over time, in response to illness progression, and the changing nature of a relationship (O'Shaughnessy *et al.* 2010; Samsi and Manthorpe 2013). The value of a relational perspective, then, is not so much in defining an 'essential nature' of decision-making (e.g. as 'individualist' or 'relational'), but is instead in enabling sensitivity to the broader range of factors that may influence how situations are appraised, and how decisions are made and enacted.

In addition to the influence of different relational coping configurations, participants also expressed how enduring values provided a frame of reference for decision-making, particularly when these decisions were unanticipated, new or complex. While autonomy and independence were valued, participants also reflected the importance of maintaining key relationships. This suggests the need to consider not only the surface features of a decision (e.g. a perceived loss of individual freedom associated with moving into residential care), but also its deeper relational significance (e.g. protecting a relationship or a symbolic 'betrayal' of trust). Thus, while transition into residential care may be perceived to be associated with a loss of independence or *individual* autonomy, in certain cases this might alternatively be interpreted as protecting and maintaining key relationships, through which ongoing *relational* autonomy is promoted. Making this interpretation requires understanding the 'trigger' for the decision, the options (or lack of options) available, and the perspectives of the different people involved (including the symbolic significance of the admission in a relational context). It also requires a sensitivity to the broader social factors (e.g. ageism and gender inequality) which have acted historically to shape peoples' beliefs of themselves as 'able and authorised' to make decisions, and which may also be an ongoing source of inequalities or undue influence in decision-making (Ho 2008; Pritchard-Jones 2017).

There are a number of limitations to this analysis, in particular the small number of cases, which precludes generalisations beyond these particular cases. However, even with a small number of cases, combining dyadic and individual interviews provided opportunities for comparisons across different social and relational situations. It could be argued that the dyadic recruitment strategy contributed to a tendency for participants to reflect more positive statements about each other to the interviewer, than they would have done if interviewed alone (Wawrziczny *et al.* 2016). While three of the cases reported here centred around the context of heterosexual couples, the single parent-child dyad yielded different perspectives, and is an important avenue for future investigation (Samsi and Manthorpe 2013). Further insights may be derived from interviews with same-sex couples and other relational configurations. Of course, caregiving relationships extend beyond partners and children, and family members also exist in reciprocal relationships with each other, leading to calls for more detailed investigation of these complex networks of family relationships and their role in decision-making (Purves and Perry 2009). Finally, these cases reveal peoples' verbal reflections on their experiences in decision-making. Other insights could be gleaned from witnessing actual decision-making in relational contexts.

## Future directions

This study has implications for future policy and practice. A recent Australian review of advance care planning among people with dementia has proposed a greater focus on understanding the person's values and beliefs; covering a broad range of issues over an extended time-period; establishing preferred substitute decision-makers; and involving the person with dementia in decision-making wherever possible (Cognitive Decline Partnership Centre 2016). Our study supports these recommendations but, additionally, would suggest that decision-making should not be understood as just an individual phenomenon, made either by the person with dementia or by a 'substitute'. A substantial number of decisions are motivated by relational concerns, and are made and enacted (or avoided) within mutually responsive relational contexts. Practitioners must promote more effective engagement with decision-making and future planning by considering the concerns of carers, and understanding the interpersonal concerns, or divergent stressor appraisals, which might lead to disputes, undue influence or one person avoiding discussions (Ho 2008). By understanding the need for decision-making as a stressor, and utilising relationally-oriented theories of stressor appraisal and coping, it may be possible to devise interventions which are better matched to people's lived experiences, and which are more effective in promoting adaptive responses within relationships, and a respectful, shared engagement with decision-making (Wawrziczny *et al.* 2016).

Practitioners can be sensitive to the relational nature of decision-making, in order to better match decision-making supports to peoples' lived experiences. At a public policy level, the recent impetus to move towards supported (as opposed to substituted) decision-making, requires a nuanced understanding of relational dynamics in decision-making, to inform the models by which decision-making support could be enacted. At a societal level, relational perspectives on decision-making alert us to some of the preconditions for the effective exercise of autonomy, including trusting relationships and supportive communication styles, and social networks for gathering information and accessing support. This suggests that autonomy is actually exercised *within* respectful, supportive relationships, and not in isolation from them. Progress in these areas will enable greater access to the social and relational platforms that provide the basis for expressing autonomy in the context of cognitive decline.

## Acknowledgements

This work was funded by the National Health and Medical Research Council and its partners in the Cognitive Decline Partnership Centre. The authors would like to acknowledge the support of these organisations and the participants who shared their experiences with the researchers.

## References

Australian Health Minister's Advisory Council, 2011, *A National Framework for Advance Care Directives.* Canberra, Australia: Australian Government Department of Health and Ageing.

Australian Institute of Health and Welfare, 2012, *Dementia in Australia*, Canberra, Australia: AIHW.

Berg, C.A., R. Upchurch, 2007, A developmental-contextual model of couples coping with chronic illness across the adult life span, *Psychological Bulletin*, 133(6): 920–954.

Berg, C.A., S.P. Meegan, F.P. Deviney, 1998, A social-contextual model of coping with everyday problems across the lifespan, *International Journal of Behavioral Development*, 22(2): 239–261.

Brannelly, T., 2011, Sustaining citizenship: People with dementia and the phenomenon of social death, *Nursing Ethics*, 18(5): 662.

Brown, M., S. Jarrad, 2008, Putting 'the powers' in place: Barriers for people with memory loss in planning for the future, *Journal of Law and Medicine*, 15(4): 530–537.

Charmaz, K., 1983, Loss of self: A fundamental form of suffering in the chronically ill, *Sociology of Health and Illness*, 5(2): 168–195.

Cognitive Decline Partnership Centre., 2016, *Future Planning and Advance Care Planning: Why it Needs to be Different for People with Dementia and Other Forms of Cognitive Decline*, https://sydney.edu.au/medicine/cdpc/documents/resources/J000606_ CDPC_report2015Final_WEB.pdf [Accessed 03 May 2018].

Dewing, J., 2007, Participatory research: A method for process consent with persons who have dementia, *Dementia*, 6(1): 11–25.

Dickinson, C., C. Bamford, C. Exley, C. Emmett, J. Hughes, L. Robinson, 2013, Planning for tomorrow whilst living for today: The views of people with dementia and their families on advance care planning, *International Psychogeriatrics*, 25(12): 2011–2021.

Epstein, R.M. 2013, Whole mind and shared mind in clinical decision-making, *Patient Education and Counseling*, 90(2): 200–206.

Fetherstonhaugh, D., L. McAuliffe, C. Shanley, M. Bauer, E. Beattie, 2017, 'Did I make the right decision?': The difficult and unpredictable journey of being a surrogate decision maker for a person living with dementia, *Dementia*, 16(6).

Fetherstonhaugh, D., L. Tarzia, R. Nay, 2013, Being central to decision making means I am still here!: The essence of decision making for people with dementia, *Journal of Aging Studies*, 27(2): 143–150.

Gooding, P., 2013, Supported decision-making: A rights-based disability concept and its implications for mental health law, *Psychiatry Psychology and Law*, 20(3): 431–451.

Gregory, R., F. Roked, L. Jones, A. Patel, 2007, Is the degree of cognitive impairment in patients with Alzheimers disease related to their capacity to appoint an enduring power of attorney?, *Age and Ageing*, 36(5): 527–531.

Gysels, M., N. Evans, A. Menaca, E. Andrew, F. Toscani, S. Finetti, P. Project, 2012, Culture and end of life care: A scoping exercise in seven European countries, *Plos One*, 7(4).

Häusler, A., A. Sánchez, P. Gellert, F. Deeken, M.A. Rapp, J. Nordheim, 2016, Perceived stress and quality of life in dementia patients and their caregiving spouses: Does dyadic coping matter? *International Psychogeriatrics*, 28(11), 1857–1866.

Hirschman, K.B., J.M. Kapo, J.H. Karlawish, 2006, Why doesn't a family member of a person with advanced dementia use a substituted judgment when making a decision for that person, *American Journal of Geriatric Psychiatry*, 14(8): 659–667.

Hirschman, K.B., J.M. Kapo, J.H.T. Karlawish, 2008, Identifying the factors that facilitate or hinder advance planning by persons with dementia, *Alzheimer Disease and Associated Disorders*, 22(3): 293–298.

Ho, A., 2008, Relational autonomy or undue pressure?: Family's role in medical decision-making, *Scandinavian Journal of Caring Sciences*, 22(1): 128–135.

Kitwood, T., 1993, Towards a theory of dementia care: The interpersonal process, *Ageing and Society*, 13(1): 51–67.

Kitwood, T., 1997, The experience of dementia, *Aging and Mental Health*, 1(1): 13–22.

Kitwood, T., K. Bredin, 1992, Towards a theory of dementia care: Personhood and well-being, *Ageing and Society*, 12(3): 269–287.

Lazarus, R., S. Folkman, 1984, *Stress, appraisal, and coping*, New York: Springer Publishing Company.

Mackenzie, C., 2008, Relational autonomy, normative authority and perfectionism, *Journal of Social Philosophy*, 39(4): 512–533.

Martin, W., S. Michalowski, T. Jutten, M. Burch, 2014, *Achieving CRPD Compliance: Is the Mental Capacity Act of England and Wales Compatible with the UN Convention on the Rights of Persons with Disabilities? If Not, What Next?*, London: University of Essex.

O'Connor, D., 2009, *Decision-Making, Personhood and Dementia: Exploring the Interface*, London: Jessica Kingsley Publishers.

O'Shaughnessy, M., K. Lee, T. Lintern, 2010, Changes in the couple relationship in dementia care: Spouse carer's experiences, *Dementia*, 9(2): 237–258.

Pritchard-Jones, L., 2017, Ageism and autonomy in health care: Explorations through a relational lens, *Health Care Analysis*, 25(1): 72–89.

Purves, B., J. Perry, 2009, Families, dementia and decision-making, in D. O'Connor, B. Purves (eds), *Decision-making, Personhood and Dementia: Exploring the Interface*, pp. 172–186, London: Jessica Kingsley Publishers.

Reamy, A. M., K. Kim, S.H. Zarit, C.J. Whitlatch, 2011, Understanding discrepancy in perceptions of values: Individuals with mild to moderate dementia and their family caregivers, *Gerontologist*, 51(4): 473–483.

Rhoden, N., 1990, The limits of legal objectivity, *North Carolina Law Review*, 68: 845–866.

Samsi, K., J. Manthorpe, 2013, Everyday decision-making in dementia: Findings from a longitudinal interview study of people with dementia and family carers, *International Psychogeriatrics*, 25(6): 949–961.

Series, L., 2015, Relationships, autonomy and legal capacity: Mental capacity and support paradigms, *Int J Law Psychiatry*, 40: 80–91.

Silvers, A., L.P. Francis, 2009, Thinking about the good: Reconfiguring liberal metaphysics (or not) for people with cognitive disabilities, *Metaphilosophy*, 40(3–4): 475–498.

Smith, J.A., P. Flowers, M. Larkin, 2009, *Interpretative Phenomenological Analysis: Theory, Method And Research*, Los Angeles, USA: Sage.

Wawrziczny, E., P. Antoine, F. Ducharme, M.J. Kergoat, F. Pasquier, 2016, Couples' experiences with early-onset dementia: An interpretative phenomenological analysis of dyadic dynamics, *Dementia-International Journal of Social Research and Practice*, 15(5): 1082–1099.

# 8 Planning for the rest-of-life, not end-of-life

## Reframing advance care planning for people with dementia

*Gail Yapp, Craig Sinclair, Adele Kelly, Kathy Williams, Ingrid Amgarth-Duff and Meera Agar*

### Background

Advance care planning (ACP) began in the United States in the 1970s and in Australia in the 1980s. It was a response to developments in medical technologies occurring from the 1960s when 'it often became difficult to distinguish saving life from prolonging suffering and death' (Sabatino 2010: 213). ACP developed out of a concern that people were receiving treatment at the end-of-life that they may not have wanted if they had been able to make their own decisions.

Historically, ACP has been aimed at extending personal autonomy, and has placed much attention on the process of completing Advance Care Directives (ACD) in which people document what it is they want or do not want for a time in the future should they be unable to make their own decisions. Most deaths in western countries occur in hospital (Broad *et al.* 2013) and medical interventions have the potential to extend the dying process while undermining dignity and the provision of comfort (Squires and Barr 2005). Hence the medical profession has been a dominant and important voice in discussions about ACP, perhaps contributing to a tendency to focus on documented ACPs, and decision-making about end-of-life medical care.

This has also meant that, in Australia where hospitals are the responsibility of State and Territory governments, a variety of approaches and legislative provisions for ACP have developed (Carter *et al.* 2016). To address this, Australia's Health Ministers recognised the need for a national policy framework, *A National Framework for Advance Care Directives* endorsed by the Australian Health Ministers' Advisory Council in 2010 (Australian Health Ministers' Advisory Council 2011). The terminology used in this chapter is based on this document, and we start by outlining what is meant by advance care planning, an advance care plan, an advanced care directive and a substitute decision-maker.

*Advance care planning (ACP):* ACP is the process of planning for future health and personal care (including lifestyle issues) where the person's values, beliefs and preferences are made known so they can guide decision-making at a future time when that person cannot make or communicate his or her decisions. ACP may be completed in a structured process with a trained professional or may occur in an informal family setting. It can include both formal and informal conversations, but does not, as we explain, always result in the recording of a person's preferences.

*Advance care plan:* Advance care plans state preferences about health and personal care and preferred health outcomes. They may be made on a person's behalf and should be prepared from the person's perspective to guide decisions about care. There are many ways of recording an advance care plan including oral and written versions. They may be made by, with or for the person. A person with diminished competence may complete an advance care plan or be assisted to complete one. A preferred decision-maker in an advance care plan is not a statutory appointment.

*Advance care directive (ACD):* An ACD is one way of formally recording an advance care plan. An ACD is one type of written advance care plan and is recognised by common law or authorised by legislation and is signed by a competent adult. An ACD can describe a person's wishes regarding their future care and can appoint a substitute decision-maker.

*Substitute decision-maker (SDM):* SDM is a term used to describe the person who is appointed or identified by law as the person able to make decisions on behalf of a person whose decision-making capacity is impaired. In this context it is used regarding the person being able to make health, medical, residential and other personal decisions. Depending on the state this person may be also termed the Enduring Attorney (Health), Enduring Guardian or Person Responsible.

The medical model of ACP, developed out of the hospital system, is characterised by a focus on the individual, and discussion is limited to medical treatment decisions and the advance documentation of a person's consent or refusal of these treatments. This approach faces a number of challenges to being adopted more broadly across the community. Major difficulties identified include a reluctance by many older people and families to discuss end-of-life issues (Rhee *et al.* 2012; Scott *et al.* 2013; Sinclair *et al.* 2014), cultural perspectives that do not align with the ideals of ACP (Shanley *et al.* 2009; Connolly *et al.* 2012; Kwak *et al.* 2014) and individuals not seeing the relevance of ACP (Schickedanz *et al.* 2009; Sinclair *et al.* 2013; Sinclair *et al.* 2014). In addition, health professionals often lack the confidence, understanding and time to discuss ACP (Shanley *et al.* 2009; Rhee *et al.* 2012; Poppe *et al.* 2013; Van der Steen *et al.* 2014). They may also be concerned that discussions about end-of-life care may erode the person's hope (Houben *et al.* 2014).

The challenges of ACP are even greater for people with dementia, given the need to develop plans well ahead of time and to review these as the illness progresses. Unfortunately, for most people, ACP is often left until it is too late for people with dementia to either initiate or be involved in these discussions (Shanley *et al.* 2009; Dening *et al.* 2011; Robinson *et al.* 2012; Poppe *et al.* 2013). Medical personnel often express concerns about the legal status of ACDs completed by people with dementia (De Boer *et al.* 2010). This means that people with dementia and other forms of cognitive decline experience barriers to ensuring their wishes are respected.

The reliability and clinical clarity of ACDs are likely to be strengthened when the ACD is discussed – or at least raised – at the time of diagnosis, or at first contact with support services. There also needs to be a pathway agreed as to how it can be reviewed regularly, ensuring it is relevant to current clinical circumstances (Carter *et al.* 2016).

Given these barriers, and the narrow focus on end-of-life decisions, it is unsurprising that awareness of ACP is low (Dickinson *et al.* 2013; Houben *et al.* 2014) and the take-up of ACDs even lower (Lewis *et al.* 2015; Sinclair *et al.* 2016). This is accentuated for those from culturally and linguistically diverse communities in which ACDs may be less culturally acceptable due to different approaches to decision-making and personal autonomy (Jeong *et al.* 2015). Additionally, in cultural contexts in which dementia is not well understood (Low *et al.* 2010; Boughtwood *et al.* 2011), dementia is more likely to be diagnosed later (Boise 2014), which in turn may reduce the opportunity for that person to participate in ACP due to the impact on cognitive capacity over time.

However, despite these challenges, there are many benefits in undertaking ACP as early as possible, for individuals, carers (informal and formal) and families of people with dementia. The benefits include improved quality of life, decreased stress and anxiety (Shanley *et al.* 2009; Rhee *et al.* 2012; Poppe *et al.* 2013; Van der Steen *et al.* 2014) and increased adherence to previously expressed wishes (Livingston *et al.* 2013). In addition, ACP assists those who will be called on to make decisions (Rhee *et al.* 2012; Shanley *et al.* 2009; Poppe *et al.* 2013; Van der Steen *et al.* 2014).

The increasing numbers of people living with dementia make it imperative that effort is made to increase early take-up of ACP for those living with this condition. In Australia, dementia is now the leading cause of disability burden for those aged 65 years or more (Australian Institute of Health and Welfare 2012) and is identified as the second leading cause of all deaths (Australian Bureau of Statistics 2015). People with dementia will make up an increasing proportion of the users of health and community care services and having an ACP in place is likely to improve outcomes. For example, when people with dementia are admitted to hospital, impairments in communication and perception, together with the change in environment and routine can cause significant distress and result in longer stays and poorer outcomes (Samaras *et al.* 2010; Sampson 2010; Australian Institute of Health and Welfare 2013), but with an ACP greater guidance for staff is likely and even the potential for hospital admission can be reduced.

## The study

Recognising the potential significant benefits of ACP for people with dementia and their carers, we undertook research to identify how to increase uptake of ACP among people with dementia. The study was funded by the Cognitive

Decline Partnership Centre and guided by an expert advisory committee. Consumers were instrumental in confirming the need for this work, and the fourth author (Williams) is a consumer representative from Dementia Australia who was on the advisory committee and also gathered and provided the perspectives of interested consumers over the course of the study.

The study sought to better understand which interventions are effective to support ACP for people with dementia by seeking the views and experience of experts and stakeholders. Participants were recruited by approaching a wide range of organisations and individuals with interest or expertise in ACP, for example, organisations representing the interests of people with dementia and carers, general practitioners and physicians who were regarded as leaders in the field of ACP, nurses and allied health workers who assisted people to complete ACP, academics who had written on the subject and government officials involved in the development and promotion of ACP. A purposive sampling framework was used to ensure participants came from a wide range of community, health and aged care settings, from consumer groups and from the different states and territories of Australia given the differing legislative and policy approaches.

Interviews were conducted over the telephone. There were 82 participants across 67 separate interviews. Most interviews were one-to-one, however, 12 organisations involved two or three participants as part of the teleconference. Of the participants, 16 came from primary care, including eight general practitioners (GPs), three practice nurses and five from primary healthcare networks; 11 came from aged care, both residential and community care; 11 from acute care; ten from ACP services operated under the auspices of hospitals in some states; eight from palliative care; eight from consumer organisations, including six from specialist dementia organisations; six from the field of geriatrics/gerontology; and six from government (including ACP policy areas and public advocates). In addition, there were three consumers (a person with dementia and two carers), two from legal areas and one from an ambulance service with involvement in ACP.

The interviews were conducted by the first (Yapp) and third (Kelly) authors. The semi-structured interviews were based on questions informed by the literature and explored barriers and enablers for ACP, and any differences in approach that were required if someone had dementia. Participants had an opportunity to ask questions and make statements regarding issues they felt were important but had not been covered. Interview length ranged from 30 to 80 minutes, with most taking 45–50 minutes. Informants from different health and aged care sectors continued to be recruited until no new themes emerged from the interviews from that particular sector.

All interviews were audio recorded and transcribed verbatim, and the transcripts were provided to participants to allow for corrections or clarifications if they wished. Around 30 per cent of the transcripts were modified by participants, primarily to clarify spoken comments into a clearer written form. Three of the interviewees made more substantial changes, providing additional information.

The transcripts were then coded using a template analysis method (King 1998), utilising NVivo (v.10) software (QSR International). In this thematic analysis, coding was based initially on an agreed structure informed by the literature, with a focus on barriers and enablers to ACP and the difference that dementia made. The themes were adapted and refined through a process of discussion by the authors Yapp and Kelly as new themes emerged from the data. The first three transcripts were dual coded independently by these authors, and differences were discussed to arrive at a common understanding. This was repeated for a further two transcripts until consistency was achieved. Authors Yapp and Kelly went through each interview at least once, and confirmed the emerging themes, with the assistance of the advisory committee.

The interviews provided a wealth of information about ACP generally. There were a number of themes, however, that are particularly relevant for people living with dementia or other forms of cognitive decline. These findings relate to the impact that the disease process has on the target group's ability to engage in ACP, their potential needs in the future and how they and their carers are treated in the health and aged care system.

## Findings

The main findings of this study in relation to ACP were that, for people with dementia: engagement with ACP needs to occur as early as possible, prior to significant loss of cognitive capacity, and that additional support may be required for continued involvement in decision-making; positive approaches focusing on how the person wishes to make the most of their life, rather than a narrow focus on medical interventions at the end-of-life are likely to be more successful; conversations, and the relationships underpinning these, are of primary importance (rather than a focus on completion of paperwork); and the appointment of a trusted SDM who knows the person with dementia well is crucial. These findings are elaborated further below, with any important differences in the setting or background of the informants highlighted.

### *Undertake ACP early to maximise meaningful participation of the person with dementia*

A number of informants from all settings identified the need to undertake ACP early for those with dementia, at a time when the ability to plan ahead was still relatively unimpaired. Informants from residential aged care settings in particular highlighted that ACP is often left too late in order for people with dementia to be meaningfully involved. This was attributed, in part, to a lack of understanding of the progressive nature of dementia. Informants from aged care, specialist dementia services and those with expertise in geriatrics/gerontology were particularly likely to raise aspects highlighting the difficulties cognitive changes had in reducing the ability to engage in ACP such as discussions about future scenarios, and to consider more abstract concepts.

The biggest difference [in ACP for people with dementia] is that we have a more limited window of catching these people. So making sure that people are introduced [to ACP] and have the opportunity to have those discussions very early on in their illness when they can still participate [is important].

(Primary care)

Specific issues to do with changes in cognition and dementia illness can change how easy it is for them [people with dementia] to engage in formalised and systemic advance care practices and also how easy it is for us as healthcare [professionals] to recognise that that's in fact what's happening.

(Palliative care)

Many of the respondents in primary care, palliative care, acute care and residential aged care settings indicated that ACP discussions often occurred with family, as the person with dementia already had reduced decision-making capacity. Encouraging ACP discussions at or soon after diagnosis of dementia, particularly in the absence of widespread take-up of ACP in the general population, is needed for people with dementia to have a greater voice into the future.

### The person with dementia is often excluded unnecessarily from decision-making

Although family involvement in decision-making can be helpful, particularly where the family or carers know and respect the views of the person with dementia, this can also have less positive outcomes. A number of informants from acute care, aged care and primary care indicated that decision-making too often relies on family decision-making to the exclusion of the person with dementia. This is not necessarily due to impaired ability. Informants indicated this was often because staff opted for an 'easier' approach, due to time pressures or lack of skills in supporting the person with dementia being involved. There were a few informants from a range of settings who spoke passionately about perceived poor outcomes due to the person with dementia's views being ignored or not sought and this was attributed to erroneous assumptions and the stigma surrounding dementia.

In particular for people with cognitive impairment I'd have to say they tend to default to the family. I've seen so many times when doctors and nurses don't even bother addressing or even looking at the person themselves just because they've got a cognitive impairment. They don't talk to the person, they talk to the family.

(Acute care)

There were some respondents, however, who indicated that people with dementia could be involved in decision-making, even very late in the disease process. These informants were from backgrounds where they had good knowledge of dementia: 'I think that persons with dementia always have a role to play in informing us in things related to their advance care planning, even to the point of people with very severe disease' (palliative care). The lack of knowledge of dementia and how people can be supported to mitigate many of the impacts excludes people from being involved in making their own decisions. It also leads to a need to consider how ACP is approached if the cognitive challenges of dementia are to be overcome.

### *Medical approaches focused on documenting wishes in respect of end-of-life limit engagement for the person with dementia*

An important component of the study was to look at the model of ACP informants were using, to determine whether there was a particular type that people with dementia were more readily able to engage with. A large proportion of respondents used a form of ACP that primarily focused on end-of-life medical issues, particularly in acute and primary care. This approach reflects the future decisions that may need to be made in these settings.

Many informants from all settings raised a number of concerns about a medical approach to ACP, particularly for people with dementia. These concerns were around focusing only on end-of-life medical interventions, completion of paperwork and the lack of certainty that still remained when decisions needed to be made. Although these issues may be relevant for all, they were particularly problematic for people with dementia. The main aspects informants raised about the traditional medical approach to ACP for people with dementia, with indicative quotes, are outlined below.

### *Problems identified in the focus on end-of-life medical interventions*

Informants, particularly from aged care, ACP services and specialist dementia services, indicated that deciding what medical interventions may or may not be wanted is difficult without a clear understanding of the diagnosis and prognosis, which is often the case with dementia. In addition, informants from specialised dementia services indicated that where there is a diagnosis, the person may be in denial regarding their condition: 'Only 50 per cent of people ever get their diagnosis of dementia and in general practice we're only just getting our heads around that and it can be at more advanced stages that they're getting diagnosed' (GP, primary care).

Understanding abstract concepts related to medical interventions was raised by some participants with expertise in dementia as a particular challenge for those with dementia. In addition, there can be difficulty imagining a future self. Informants indicated that the impact of dementia on a person's ability to plan, understand/have insight and make decisions means that the likelihood of engaging with ACP will decrease as the condition progresses. Those from aged care indicated there was often a lack of understanding of what the potential medical interventions meant.

By the time that families start to realise that things are going wrong, it's often too late for them to participate ... the person finds it very hard to grasp the concepts that you are trying to get them to think about.

(Gerontologist)

Informants from all settings indicated that a focus on end-of-life means that staff, family and the person with dementia often find the subject of ACP too confronting to raise. This is compounded because of the range of 'bad news' that often accompanies dementia and the stigma surrounding it: 'Doctors do not feel comfortable talking about [ACP] ... the doctors just don't bring up the subject' (aged care). Some informants from consumer groups in particular indicated that there are other issues that may be of greater concern to people than end-of-life issues. These can include ensuring important aspects to the person such as faith and culture are respected, and having some say in what might happen in the future around care and accommodation as the condition progresses.

It's not just about medical treatment, it might be [about planning] where someone's going to be cared for, or who they're going to be cared for by, or what kinds of things or activities do people still want to participate in.

(Carer/consumer group)

*Problems identified with a focus on completion of paperwork*

Across all settings participants, but particularly specialist ACP services, indicated that people are often very reluctant to commit their views in writing. There was a preference for discussions and informal plans over formally documenting wishes. People are also concerned about the ability to change ACDs if their perspectives change in the future. Formal ACDs can be changed in all jurisdictions, but the fear remains, and a diagnosis of dementia may contribute to this if there is concern about future capacity.

Many participants indicated that documents completed without expert assistance may be confusing, particularly where they deal with medical terminology.

The patient finds them [ACDs] very distressing to fill in, and so do the families, because there's a lot of specifics in there ... they get really confused about what situations to put 'yes' and what to put 'no' to.

(Primary care)

The other thing that has been a bit of barrier ... is that people are required to list treatments that they do or do not want in advance and that's really difficult for lay people to do. Most people would know what quality of life means to them, but how do you document the CPR decision ... [and] other kinds of health decisions that come along when you've got dementia or other kinds of co-morbidity.

(Carer/consumer group)

Many respondents from across a range of settings also indicated that written ACDs were often ignored or could not be found when needed. They may be ignored by family members who are not in agreement with them, or by medical staff who are not aware of their legal standing. Informants advised that on completion, they may often be put in a drawer, lost in the depths of a patient's file or kept in a doctor's or lawyer's office which means they are not available out of hours.

> My personal opinion is that pieces of paper are helpful but they're not the 'be all and end all', they're not what you live and die by because, at the end of the day, a piece of paper can be ripped up, it can be disregarded, it can be questioned, … it can also hold people back from having treatment which actually could be very effective for them … The piece of paper is a reminder that you've had that conversation and it can be a memory prompt.
>
> (Acute care)

> There's very good evidence that doctors will be influenced by such documents [ACDs] if they can be found. Although as you are probably aware, it's rare for them to be available at the time when decisions need to be made.
>
> (Acute care)

*Documents completed ahead of time may not provide the certainty and authority medical staff require*

Participants in acute care settings and from the government expressed concern about the clarity, reliability and currency of ACP documents, and a lack of certainty about applicability to the current situation: 'The most common comment is "these things aren't worth the paper they're written on". I must have had that said to me a hundred times this year so far' (acute care).

Some participants indicated that medical personnel would prefer to have documents completed only at the time of an admission or by the person's doctor.

> The MOLST [Medical Orders for Life Sustaining Treatment] becomes a legal document because it's a medical order … So it's not an advance care directive. It's a medical order for life sustaining treatment and because it's signed off by everyone and the doctor at the hospital can see that the GP has been involved and the health professional has been involved and the family are on board, they're much more likely to follow it.
>
> (Aged care)

On the other hand, this approach of making decisions at the time of an acute event or hospital admission means that a person with dementia is less able to initiate these requirements, and there is reliance on the family or person's doctor to know their wishes and have these incorporated into the decision-making.

**Focusing on discussions and understanding values and wishes for the rest-of-life, within the context of relationships, is more likely to be successful**

Participants who regularly facilitate ACP described the benefits of a broader psychosocial approach, focusing more on the identification of values, the importance of conversations about a wide variety of topics and strengthening relationships. The focus should be on understanding what is valued and important to the person so that future decisions can be informed by these. These types of conversations were considered by many informants to be more positive, making it easier for the person with dementia, their family and for staff.

*Focusing on a person's values can inform decision-making*

Participants indicated that if the person's values and ideals are understood then decisions can be informed by these values in any given situation because values are less subject to change and rely less on the person's medical knowledge. There is a need to move from a focus on formal documentation to one focused on values, engagement and conversation between all parties (Siddiqui 2016).

> Ideally advance care planning … should be targeted towards a person's goals and we shouldn't make it their responsibility to say, 'yes I want this, no I don't want that' in a shopping list sort of way … [We should be] understanding the person's goals and then fitting healthcare options to those goals rather than making people choose between the big shopping list by themselves.
>
> (Palliative care)

*The importance of engagement with family as part of the process*

Having people make decisions in advance, without considering family and others around them, was raised by informants as an important barrier to ACP. An approach to autonomy which better recognises that people make decisions in the context of relationships, family and culture may create greater engagement with ACP and reduce later conflict when decisions need to be made. It also better recognises the approach taken to decision-making in many culturally diverse communities.

> People aren't these rugged individuals that go around writing documents about their care. They are social people who are concerned about the implications of their decisions for their family and they tend to want to make them together with their family. How that's documented is probably less important than the process that they go through.
>
> (Acute care)

*Focusing on how a person wants to live not how they want to die*

Participants from community and aged care settings noted that discussions about what the person considers important are easier for family or staff members to raise, and easier for a person with some cognitive loss to engage with. It was also felt that conversations were more positive and affirming if they focus on living rather than dying.

*Importance of discussion of a wide variety of topics*

Some participants, particularly in community and aged care settings, observed that people live with dementia for an extended period of time, and face many lifestyle decisions as well as care and health decisions as the condition progresses. This includes decisions about pets and visitors, retirement from driving, location of care and living arrangements as well as decisions about medications or medical interventions. For people in rural or regional areas, informants indicated there is often a desire to remain close to family or community, even if this limits what care is available. Examples were also given for those with younger onset dementia where there are also considerations about work and children.

> There's a whole lot of decisions … do you downsize, do you move, do you want to live with your family or not, what are the things you might need to take into account, what do you like doing, what do you want to keep doing as much as possible. Having the discussion around what's important to you, and therefore end of life issues and preferences are just part of conversation.
>
> (Aged care)

> If I went to a doctor, the doctor would just be focused on the medical treatment side and they wouldn't be thinking about my dress standards or grooming or the kind of things that give my life meaning.
>
> (Carer/consumer organisation)

*Encouraging conversations*

The conversations that occur in the context of personal relationships were considered the most important aspect of ACP for many respondents. The conversations mean that a range of issues can be explored in a natural way and family and SDMs understand how the person approaches decision-making and their underlying values and what they consider most important.

> So it's really that people relationship, it comes back to that. I think that's at the heart of advance care planning anyway. It's about conversations, about people, it's about relationships – that's what it's fundamentally all about, and that's what works best for us as well.
>
> (ACP service)

The social environment in which people operate, how they take into consideration the implications for others, and whether they prefer to make decisions together or after discussion, are all important relational issues identified by participants.

> The conversation is such a major part of the whole journey of advance care planning. It's something that is vital. ... We need to have people having these discussions regardless even of any documents being completed.
>
> (ACP service)

> We've got no way of knowing how many people actually go through and complete the process, but in some ways, I'm not sure that that matters. That's the icing on the cake if you like, and that's what I say to community groups when I talk to them and to service providers. I say, the cake is the conversation, the icing on the cake is completing the documentation, but the cake is actually the conversation.
>
> (Palliative care)

### Appointment of a SDM is crucial

Across all settings and models of ACP one area of agreed importance was the value of appointing a trusted SDM. Two areas were highlighted as important: appointing an appropriate person who understands one's wishes and the support and knowledge a SDM needs to undertake the role effectively.

### Importance of appointing a trusted person

A well-chosen SDM – through a legal enduring guardian approach or through ACP – was widely regarded across community and aged care settings as critical to good outcomes. This was because it was felt that the SDM must have the capacity to be an active advocate for the person to receive care consistent with their wishes. It was felt that for people from culturally and linguistically diverse backgrounds, it is important for the SDM to have an understanding of the person's culture.

> Probably the most critical element is the medical enduring power of attorney and making sure that that power of attorney knows what that person would want.
>
> (Aged care)

> Who you choose [as a SDM] is really important. I do talk to people about what kind of characteristics I think people need like clear headedness, a level of assertiveness, and an ability to be calm, ... but most importantly I say they are your voice. If they can't speak for you without their own values and preferences and wishes and ideas about what they think is best for you getting in the way, then they're not the person you should be nominating.
>
> (Palliative care)

*Knowledge, understanding and discussion is important*

Participants across all settings identified the importance of good conversations with SDMs and family, rather than a reliance on completion of documents. Conversations were considered fundamental to planning in advance and the SDM being able to make the decision the person would have made.

> It's about person-centred care at the end of the day isn't it? So if you have expressed wishes, if you have discussed it with your substitute decision maker and they know what your values are and what's important to you then you're more likely to get person-centred care or likely to get care that accords with your wishes and values as an individual.
>
> (Aged care)

*Support is needed so that SDMs undertake their role effectively*

The difficulty for families in making decisions on behalf of a person with dementia was highlighted in personal stories provided by participants who express the anxiety and ongoing discomfort with decisions made many years previously. A number of informants from aged care and acute care indicated that families and SDMs do not always understand their role – that they should be seeking to consider what the person would want rather than what they want for themselves. This can be compounded when there is family conflict. The informants indicated greater support was needed so that SDMs understood they were making a decision on behalf of the person. Informants from aged care highlighted the benefit of talking with SDMs ahead of time so that decisions could be well informed and considered, rather than just a reaction in an emergency.

> I think it is a huge barrier for health professionals to be having an advance directive but then to have a family member sitting there going, 'you've got to treat, you've got to treat' and just ignore everything they have said. It's a huge barrier.
>
> (Consumer)

> We are seeing an increase, a slow but steady increase in conflict in this setting and we really have to do far more to try and shore up our understanding of what the patient themselves actually want because in the end that's always the circuit breaker.
>
> (Specialist, acute care)

## Discussion

The findings from this study of the views and experience of a wide range of informants have important implications for how ACP is best approached in order  to encourage greater adoption for people with dementia and their carers.

The study findings highlight the need to address the difficulties of medically focused ACP and to frame ACP within the context of encouraging relational autonomy, particularly for those with dementia.

### *Relational autonomy is considered to be very important*

The progressive impact of dementia on cognitive ability means that over time the person will find it more difficult to make their own decisions and to care for themselves. It has been argued that a sense of connectedness and being in an affirming relationship with others is a vital contributor to quality of life for people with dementia (Kitwood 1997; Nolan *et al.* 2004; Morhardt and Spira 2013; Sabat 2014; O'Rourke *et al.* 2015). Concern for family is a key motivator for older people (Levi *et al.* 2010) and people with dementia (Dening *et al.* 2013). An ACP which incorporates such values could help to alleviate this distress for both people living with dementia and their family members.

Participants in the research study widely supported a values-based discussion to strengthen the knowledge transfer to future decision-makers. This entails a move from the individualist conception of autonomy inherent in a medical approach, to one which better recognises the importance of relationships and the role of family carers (Whitlatch and Menne 2009; Pollard 2015). This approach is also likely to be more acceptable to those from culturally and linguistically diverse communities (Searight and Gafford 2005; Bullock 2011; Ekore and Lanre-Abass 2016; Siddiqui 2016).

Moving towards a values-based approach is also supported by the literature (Prommer 2010; Sinclair *et al.* 2016). A focus on identifying values and what is important to the person which can occur in informal discussions can mean that some of the barriers to ACP for those with dementia are overcome, including the reluctance or avoidance of people engaging in ACP discussions, and not finding the 'right' time to initiate ACP discussions, with subsequent loss of capacity (Brooke and Kirk 2014).

Strengthening the understanding of a person's values and preferences through a relational approach to ACP can be very helpful to SDMs in making the multitude of decisions that need to be made on behalf of the person with dementia. Where the focus includes an understanding of how decisions were approached and priorities, it can aid SDMs in making decisions about care (such as respite and residential care) as well as end-of-life care (Reamy *et al.* 2011).

### *Addressing the difficulties of medically focused ACP*

Informants from all settings identified a range of barriers to medically focused ACP. The focus on determining an individual's wishes in relation to end-of-life medical interventions and reliance on completion of documents limits engagement with ACP. While this model of ACP has meant there have been resources available to develop and encourage consideration of end-of-life medical issues, this narrow approach has many significant shortcomings and is even less effective and appropriate for people with dementia (McMahan *et al.* 2013). It is difficult for a person to predict preferences for specific interventions without the lived experience. The value of someone in a trusted relationship raising and encouraging ACP has been recognised in other studies (Briggs 2004; Rhee *et al.* 2013; Van der Steen *et al.* 2014). The potential role that a reframed approach to ACP could play in improving both engagement and decision-making for the benefit of people with dementia, their families and SDMs comes from the literature on dementia care where the benefits of a person-centred or psychosocial approach are highlighted, often in contrast with a medical model where the focus is on individuals and loss of functioning (Fazio 2013; Williams *et al.* 2014).

The suggestion from informants, that ACP needs to cover a much broader range of issues in recognition of the extended period of time in which people with dementia may not have the capacity to make their own decisions, has only limited coverage in the literature. Participation in research (Dowson *et al.* 2013; Nuffield Council on Bioethics 2009) and retirement from driving (Carmody *et al.* 2013) are other non-medical issues that have been identified as benefiting from inclusion in ACP.

Proxy decision-making can often be distressing for families (Lord *et al.* 2015). ACP relieves the stress on family members and SDMs (Detering *et al.* 2010; Chiarchiaro *et al.* 2015) and this is used to encourage take-up. Family and SDMs of those with dementia face a large number of decisions over the course of the disease and decisions other than end-of-life ones may cause greater stress, in particular placement in residential care (Elliott *et al.* 2009; Livingston *et al.* 2010; Koplow *et al.* 2015; Lord *et al.* 2015; Webb and Dening 2016). The greatest distress for family and SDMs is when decisions are made that seem to be in conflict with what the person themselves might have wanted, and where they do not have support from healthcare professionals (Lord *et al.* 2015). Family members, particularly spouses, often agonise over residential care placement, and yet people with dementia are often concerned about their family carer's wellbeing and may be more open to a move than others have realised (Whitlatch and Menne 2009).

Where family understand the person with dementia's values and preferences, this leads to greater involvement of the person with dementia in decision-making (Miller *et al.* 2016). It also can reduce decisional conflict for proxy decision-makers by having values inform treatment rather than providing firm indications about specific treatments (Kwak *et al.* 2015). In the development of a two-question ACD (Mahon 2011) that is non-threatening, encouraged discussion and recognised the uncertainties of future care, Mahon argued that 'at their best, advance directives comprise two components: designation of a surrogate decision maker and identification of factors and preferences to guide decision making' (2011: 803).

## *Future directions for practice, research and policy*

This research demonstrates that a more positive and personal approach to ACP is likely to achieve greater success in engaging people with dementia and their families. Such an approach removes the barriers to ACP inherent in a medical approach focused on end-of-life, instead focusing on the matters that people with dementia and their families consider the most important. A focus on values and what has guided and informed decisions in the past also overcomes the difficulty many people with dementia have in envisaging a future self (De Boer *et al.* 2012). The priority for health and aged care professionals will be to encourage a person with dementia to appoint a trusted person to make decisions on their behalf in the future and to have discussions with them so that they know what is most valued. An ACD might also be promoted, particularly in situations where someone wishes to formalise their choices for medical care in the future, or where there is no close family member.

The findings also highlight other areas that need to be considered in relation to how decision-making is put into place and the supports that people with dementia, their families and SDMs may need. A person with dementia should be included in decision-making as far as possible, and for as long as possible. SDMs may also need support to understand their role in making the decision that the person with dementia is likely to have made if they had been able to, rather than the decision they would wish for. Encouraging a broader scope for advance planning may mean that the person with dementia raises issues which are outside the scope of practice of health professionals. This will mean that health professionals will need to develop good relationships and links with stakeholders who can support other planning/decisions if outside their knowledge, and provide guidance to the person with dementia and their family about how to find support in this area. A broader approach to ACP also provides opportunities for those in the community aged care sector to work more closely with people with dementia and their carers in identifying 'care values' (Whitlatch 2013, 2014) to strengthen relationships and inform consumer-directed care packages.

The amount of research in relation to ACP has grown significantly in recent years and the specific issues in relation to those with dementia have also emerged only relatively recently. However, this work has been primarily based on the issues related to end-of-life medical care rather than considering how best to encourage planning for a broader range of issues likely to be of concern for people with dementia, their SDMs and families. Research into how to support the consideration of decisions other than end-of-life care are still in the early stages and to date show mixed results (Sampson *et al.* 2011; Lord *et al.* 2015, 2016). Further research is needed to identify the areas of most concern to people living with dementia and families in considering the future and how best to incorporate this into future planning that already occurs or could be supported in a range of settings.

In order to make the ACP process more relevant for people with dementia and their families and SDMs there is a need to reframe it as one which allows consideration of the broad range of issues of importance to people with dementia and for which decisions will need to be made over the remaining period of life. This will require greater consideration of whether the range of structures established to support ACP are appropriate for the increasing proportion of older people with dementia in the community. This will include looking at prescribed or suggested forms, the settings in which assistance is provided and the messages conveyed by medical practitioners at diagnosis, support workers, online or in promotional campaigns. It is encouraging to see that South Australia, the Australian jurisdiction who has most recently reviewed their approach to ACP, has put in place an ACD form which explicitly covers a broad range of issues and supports a person being able to indicate what is of importance to them and what should be considered in making decisions for them (Department of Health and Ageing and GOSA 2016).

The other important area to better address through policy is in relation to decision-making for those with impaired cognitive abilities. There are three aspects that are likely to benefit greatly from improved support: (a) providing guidance on the wise choice of SDMs as part of ACP; (b) supporting a person to be involved in decision-making for as long as possible, including through supported decision-making; and (c) providing assistance to SDMs to better understand their role. Given the key role SDMs play in the lives of people with dementia, and their unpreparedness for this role, there may be value in seeking to increase engagement with ACP and discussions of values to inform advance planning through specifically targeting family members who may be SDMs in the future.

Our research clearly indicates that the medical model of ACP with its focus on health interventions is not working, particularly for those with dementia. The solutions identified fit within a person-centred and social model with a focus on relationships. This points to the need for informed discussions to identify what is important to the person or most valued, the appointment of trusted substitute decision-makers who know the person well, supporting a person to be involved with decision-making as much as possible and planning how best to live the rest-of-life by considering a broad range of issues.

Future action should focus on planning ahead on a wide range of issues, including what actions can be taken to reduce the impact of disability; the importance of appointing a SDM, including how to choose; and encouraging conversations with SDMs and family on what is most valued. Achieving greater engagement with ACP for those living with dementia will mean they are more likely to receive care and support in line with their wishes, increasing their quality of life. SDMs, carers and family will benefit too, knowing that the decisions that need to be made reflect the values and wishes of the person they love and care for.

## Acknowledgements

This work was funded by the National Health and Medical Research Council and its partners in the Cognitive Decline Partnership Centre. The generosity with time and ideas of those interviewed is greatly appreciated – this paper aims to ensure their perspectives are more broadly available.

## References

Australian Bureau of Statistics, 2015, *Causes of Death, Australia*, http://www.abs.gov.au/ ausstats/abs@.nsf/Lookup/by%20Subject/3303.0~2015~Main%20Features~ Australia's%20leading%20causes%20of%20death,%202015~3.

Australian Health Ministers' Advisory Council, 2011, *A National Framework for Advance Care Directives*, www.ahmac.gov.au.

Australian Institute of Health and Welfare, 2012, *Dementia in Australia*, Canberra, Australia: AIHW.

Australian Institute of Health and Welfare, 2013, *Dementia Care in Hospitals: Costs and Strategies*, Canberra, Australia: AIHW.

Boise, L., 2014, Ethnicity and dementia, in M. Downs and B. Bowers (eds), *Excellence in Dementia Care: Research Into Practice*, pp. 36–52, Maidenhead, UK: McGraw-Hill Education (UK).

Bollig, G., E. Gjengedal, J.H. Rosland, 2016, They know!–Do they?: A qualitative study of residents and relatives views on advance care planning, end-of-life care, and decision-making in nursing homes, *Palliative Medicine*, 30: 456–470.

Boughtwood, D., C. Shanley, J. Adams, Y. Santalucia, H. Kyriazopoulos, D. Pond, J. Rowland, 2011, Culturally and linguistically diverse (CALD) families dealing with dementia: An examination of the experiences and perceptions of multicultural community link workers, *Journal of Cross-Cultural Gerontology*, 26: 365–377.

Briggs, L., 2004, Shifting the focus of advance care planning: Using an in-depth interview to build and strengthen relationships, *Journal of Palliative Medicine*, 7: 341–349.

Broad, J.B., M. Gott, H. Kim, M. Boyd, H. Chen, M.J. Connolly, 2013, Where do people die?: An international comparison of the percentage of deaths occurring in hospital and residential aged care settings in 45 populations, using published and available statistics, *International Journal of Public Health*, 58: 257–267.

Brooke, J., M. Kirk, 2014, Advance care planning for people living with dementia, *British Journal of Community Nursing*, 19.

Bullock, K., 2011, The influence of culture on end-of-life decision making, *Journal of Social Work in End-of-Life & Palliative Care*, 7: 83–98.

Carmody, J., V. Traynor, D. Iverson, E. Marchetti, 2013, Driving, dementia and Australian physicians: Primum non nocere?, *Internal Medicine Journal*, 43: 625–630.

Carter, R.Z., K.M. Detering, W. Silvester, E. Sutton, 2016, Advance care planning in Australia: What does the law say?, *Australian Health Review*, 40: 405–414.

Chiarchiaro, J., P. Buddadhumaruk, R.M. Arnold, D.B. White, 2015, Prior advance care planning is associated with less decisional conflict among surrogates for critically ill patients, *Annals of the American Thoracic Society*, 12: 1528–1533.

Connolly, A., E.L. Sampson, N. Purandare, 2012, End-of-life care for people with dementia from ethnic minority groups: A systematic review, *Journal American Geriatric Society*, 60: 351–360.

De Boer, M.E., C.M. Hertogh, R.M. Droes, C. Jonker, J.A. Eefsting, 2010, Advance directives in dementia: Issues of validity and effectiveness, *International Psychogeriatrics*, 22: 201–208.

De Boer, M.E., R-M Dröes, C. Jonker, J.A. Eefsting, C.M. Hertogh, 2012, Thoughts on the future: The perspectives of elderly people with early-stage Alzheimer's disease and the implications for advance care planning, *AJOB Primary Research*, 3: 14–22.

Dening, K.H., L. Jones, E.L. Sampson, 2011, Advance care planning for people with dementia: A review, *International Psychogeriatrics*, 23: 1535–1551.

Dening, K.H., L. Jones, E.L. Sampson, 2013, Preferences for end-of-life care: A nominal group study of people with dementia and their family carers, *Palliative Medicine*, 27: 409–417.

Department of Health and Ageing (DOHA), GOSA, 2016, Advance care directive DIY kit – Making your future health and life choices known, *Current ACD Guide*, https:// advancecaredirectives.sa.gov.au/upload/home/Current_ACD_Guide.pdf.

Detering, K.M., A.D. Hancock, M.C. Reade, W. Silvester, 2010, The impact of advance care planning on end of life care in elderly patients: Randomised controlled trial, *BMJ*, 340: c1345.

Dickinson, C., C. Bamford, C. Exley, C. Emmett, J. Hughes, L. Robinson, 2013, Planning for tomorrow whilst living for today: The views of people with dementia and their families on advance care planning, *International Psychogeriatrics*, 25: 2011–2021.

Dowson, L., C. Doyle, V. Rayner, 2013, Scoping the ethics of dementia research within an Australian human research context, *Journal of Law and Medicine*, 21: 210–216.

Ekore, R.I., B. Lanre-Abass, 2016, African cultural concept of death and the idea of advance care directives, *Indian Journal of Palliative Care*, 22: 369.

Elliott, B.A., C.E. Gessert, C. Peden-Mcalpine, 2009, Family decision-making in advanced dementia: Narrative and ethics, *Scand J Caring Science*, 23: 251–258.

Fazio, S., 2013, The individual is the core—and the key—to the person centered care, *Generations*, 37: 16–22.

Houben, C.H., M.A. Spruit, M.T. Groenen, E.F. Wouters, D.J. Janssen, 2014, Efficacy of advance care planning: A systematic review and meta-analysis. *J Am Med Dir Assoc*, 15: 477–489.

Jeong, S., S. Ohr, J. Pich, P. Saul, A. Ho, 2015, 'Planning ahead' among community-dwelling older people from culturally and linguistically diverse background: A cross-sectional survey, *Journal of Clinical Nursing*, 24: 244–255.

King, N., 1998, Template analysis, in G.E. Symon and C.E. Casell (eds), *Qualitative Methods and Analysis in Organizational Research: A Practical Guide*, pp. 118–134, Thousand Oaks, USA: Sage Publications Ltd.

Kitwood, T., 1997, *Dementia Reconsidered: The Person Comes First*, Buckingham, UK: Open University Press.

Koplow, S.M., A.M. Gallo, K.A. Knafl, C. Vincent, O. Paun, V. Gruss, 2015, Family caregivers define and manage the nursing home placement process, *Journal of Family Nursing*, 21: 469–493.

Kwak, J., J.A. De Larwelle, T. Kesler, 2015, Role of advance care planning in proxy decision making among individuals with dementia and their family caregivers, *Research in Gerontological Nursing*, 9: 72–80.

Kwak, J., E. Ko, B.J. Kramer, 2014, Facilitating advance care planning with ethnically diverse groups of frail, low-income elders in the USA: Perspectives of care managers on challenges and recommendations, *Health and Social Care in the Community*, 22: 169–177.

Levi, B.H., C. Dellasega, M. Whitehead, M.J. Green, 2010, What influences individuals to engage in advance care planning?, *Am J Hosp Palliat Care*, 27: 306–312.

Lewis, M., E. Rand, E. Mullaly, D. Mellor, S. Macfarlane, 2015, Uptake of a newly implemented advance care planning program in a dementia diagnostic service, *Age and Ageing*, 44: 1045–1049.

Livingston, G., G. Leavey, M. Manela, D. Livingston, G. Rait, E. Sampson, S. Bavishi, K. Shahriyarmolki, C. Cooper, 2010, Making decisions for people with dementia who lack capacity: Qualitative study of family carers in UK, *BMJ*, 341: c4184.

Livingston, G., E. Lewis-Holmes, C. Pitfield, M. Manela, D. Chan, E. Constant, H. Jacobs, G. Wills, N. Carson, J. Morris, 2013, Improving the end-of-life for people with dementia living in a care home: An intervention study, *International Psychogeriatrics*, 25(11): 1849–1858.

Lord, K., G. Livingston, C. Cooper, 2015, A systematic review of barriers and facilitators to and interventions for proxy decision-making by family carers of people with dementia, *International Psychogeriatrics*, 27: 1301–1312.

Lord, K., G. Livingston, S. Robertson, C. Cooper, 2016, How people with dementia and their families decide about moving to a care home and support their needs: Development of a decision aid, a qualitative study, *BMC Geriatrics*, 16: 68.

Low, L-F, K.J. Anstey, S.M. Lackersteen, M. Camit, F. Harrison, B. Draper, H. Brodaty, 2010, Recognition, attitudes and causal beliefs regarding dementia in Italian, Greek and Chinese Australians, *Dementia and Geriatric Cognitive Disorders*, 30: 499–508.

Mahon, M.M., 2011, An advance directive in two questions, *Journal of Pain and Symptom Management*, 41: 801–807.

McMahan, R.D., S.J. Knight, T.R. Fried, R.L. Sudore, 2013, Advance care planning beyond advance directives: Perspectives from patients and surrogates, *Journal of Pain and Symptom Management*, 46: 355–365.

Miller, L.M., C.J. Whitlatch, K.S. Lyons, 2016, Shared decision-making in dementia: A review of patient and family carer involvement, *Dementia*, 15: 1141–1157.

Morhardt, D., M. Spira, 2013, From person-centered care to relational centered care, *Generations*, 37: 37–44.

Nolan, M.R., S. Davies, J. Brown, J. Keady, J. Nolan, 2004, Beyond 'person-centred' care: A new vision for gerontological nursing, *Journal of Clinical Nursing*, 13: 45–53.

Nuffield Council on Bioethics., 2009, *Dementia: Ethical issues*, London: Nuffield Council on Bioethics.

O'Rourke, H.M., W. Duggleby, K.D. Fraser, L. Jerke, 2015, Factors that affect quality of life from the perspective of people with dementia: A metasynthesis, *Journal of the American Geriatrics Society*, 63, 24–38.

Pollard, C.L., 2015, What is the right thing to do: Use of a relational ethic framework to guide clinical decision-making, *International Journal of Caring Sciences*, 8: 362–368.

Poppe, M., S. Burleigh, S. Banerjee, 2013, Qualitative evaluation of advanced care planning in early dementia (ACP-ED), *PLoS One*, 8: e60412.

Prommer, E.E., 2010, Using the values-based history to fine-tune advance care planning for oncology patients, *Journal of Cancer Education*, 25: 66–69.

Reamy, A.M., K. Kim, S.H. Zarit, C.J. Whitlatch, 2011, Understanding discrepancy in perceptions of values: Individuals with mild to moderate dementia and their family caregivers, *The Gerontologist*, 51: 473–483.

Rhee, J.J., N.A. Zwar, L.A. Kemp, 2012, Uptake and implementation of Advance Care Planning in Australia: Findings of key informant interviews, *Aust Health Rev*, 36: 98–104.

Rhee, J.J., N.A. Zwar, L.A. Kemp, 2013, Advance care planning and interpersonal relationships: A two-way street, *Family Practice*, 30: 219–226.

Robinson, L., C. Dickinson, N. Rousseau, F. Beyer, A. Clark, J. Hughes, D. Howel, C. Exley, 2012, A systematic review of the effectiveness of advance care planning interventions for people with cognitive impairment and dementia, *Age and Ageing*, 41: 263–269.

Sabat, S.R, 2014, A bio-psycho-social approach to dementia, in M. Downs and B. Bowers (eds), *Excellence in Dementia Care: Research Into Practice*, pp, 107–121, London: McGraw-Hill Education.

Sabatino, C.P, 2010, The evolution of health care advance planning law and policy, *The Milbank Quarterly*, 88: 211–239.

Samaras, N., T. Chevalley, D. Samaras, G. Gold, 2010, Older patients in the emergency department: A review, *Annals of emergency medicine*, 56: 261–269.

Sampson, E.L., 2010, Palliative care for people with dementia, *British Medical Bulletin*, 96: 159–174.

Sampson, E.L., L. Jones, I.C. Thune-Boyle, R. Kukkastenvehmas, M. King, B. Leurent, A. Tookman, M.R. Blanchard, 2011, Palliative assessment and advance care planning in severe dementia: An exploratory randomized controlled trial of a complex intervention, *Palliative Medicine*, 25: 197–209.

Schickedanz, A.D., D. Schillinger, C.S. Landefeld, S.J. Knight, B.A. Williams, R.L. Sudore, 2009, A clinical framework for improving the advance care planning process: Start with patients' self-identified barriers, *J Am Geriatr Soc*, 57: 31–39.

Scott, I.A., G.K. Mitchell, E.J. Reymond, M.P. Daly, 2013, Difficult but necessary conversations: The case for advance care planning, *Med J Aust*, 199: 662–666.

Searight, H.R., J. Gafford, 2005, Cultural diversity at the end of life: Issues and guidelines for family physicians, *American family physician*, 71.

Shanley, C., E. Whitmore, A. Khoo, C. Cartwright, A. Walker, R.G. Cumming, 2009, Understanding how advance care planning is approached in the residential aged care setting: A continuum model of practice as an explanatory device, *Australasian Journal on Ageing*, 28: 211–215.

Siddiqui, S., 2016, Ethical challenges facing advance care planning, *Asian Bioethics Review*, 8: 53–65.

Sinclair, C., J. Smith, Y. Toussaint, K. Auret, 2013, Discussing dying in the diaspora: Attitudes towards advance care planning among first generation Dutch and Italian migrants in rural Australia, *Social Science & Medicine*, 101: 86–93.

Sinclair, C., G. Williams, A. Knight, K. Auret, 2014, A public health approach to promoting advance care planning to Aboriginal people in regional communities, *Australian Journal of Rural Health*, 22: 23–28.

Sinclair, J.B., J.R. Oyebode, R.G. Owens, 2016, Consensus views on advance care planning for dementia: A Delphi study, *Health & Social Care in the Community*, 24: 165–174.

Squires, B., F. Barr, 2005, The development of advance care directives in New South Wales, *Australasian Journal on Ageing*, 24.

Van Der Steen, J.T., M.C. Van Soest-Poortvliet, M. Hallie-Heierman, B.D. Onwuteaka-Philipsen, L. Deliens, M.E. De Boer, L. Van Den Block, N. Van Uden, C.M. Hertogh, H.C. De Vet, 2014, Factors associated with initiation of Advance Care Planning in dementia: A systematic review, *J Alzheimers Dis*, 40: 743–757.

Webb, R., K.H. Dening, 2016, In whose best interests?: A case study of a family affected by dementia, *British Journal of Community Nursing*, 21.

Whitlatch, C., 2013, Person-centered care in the early stages of dementia: Honoring individuals and their choices, *Generations*, 37: 30–36.

Whitlatch, C., 2014, Understanding and enhancing the relationship between people with dementia and their family carers, in M. Downs and B. Bowers (eds), *Excellence in Dementia Care: Research Into Practice*, London: McGraw-Hill Education.

Whitlatch, C., H. Menne, 2009, Don't forget about me!: Decision making by people with dementia, *Generations*, 33: 66–73.

Williams, B.R., T.L. Blizard, P.S. Goode, C.N. Harada, L.L. Woodby, K.L. Burgio, R. Sims, 2014, Exploring the affective dimension of the life review process: Facilitators' interactional strategies for fostering personhood and social value among older adults with early dementia, *Dementia*, 13: 498–524.

# Part III

# Persons in relationship

The dynamics of care

Part II

Persons in relationships

# 9 The critical importance of adopting a 'personhood lens' in reframing support and care for those with dementia

*Lynette R. Goldberg, Andrea D. Price, Susanne E. Becker and Aidan Bindoff*

## Introduction[1]

This chapter focuses on an online dementia education programme that has, as its core theoretical base, a social model of care. The authors share their experiences of students learning to adopt this relationship-based approach in one particular unit of the programme. Students in this unit were primarily those paid to support and care for people with dementia, admitted to hospital or residing in an aged care community. An analysis of students' comments documented their insight into the importance of person-centred care and their ability to build on their previous experience and knowledge to fold a person-centred approach into socially-engaged and dignity-preserving care for people with dementia. Further, students recognised the need to attend to the valuable experiences, knowledge and voices of those who provide care, both paid and unpaid, to optimise quality of life for all in any caring relationship.

Dementia is a multi-faceted syndrome, and recognised as a global public health issue (Prince *et al.* 2015). Although the risk of developing dementia increases with age, this progressive, neurological, life-changing and life-limiting condition is not a normal part of ageing (World Health Organization 2012). Concerns about the possibility of dementia arise when there are changes in a person's memory, sustained attention, processing speed, visuospatial skills, word finding ability, personality or mood and behaviour. Daily functional activities likely to be affected include driving, cooking, taking prescribed medications correctly, operating the television remote control, emailing, using the telephone, sleeping, managing finances, making decisions, navigating and being confident in social situations (Slavin *et al.* 2013). As people move along the dementia trajectory, these changes may have profound and adverse effects on their ability to function independently and lead to increasing reliance on care from family members or paid caregivers (Marventano *et al.* 2015; Nikmat *et al.* 2015). To optimise quality of life, such care needs to focus on the unique needs and social engagement of each individual (Macdonald 2018). To understand these individual needs and provide connected and socially-engaged care, a 'personhood lens' is essential.

## Person-centred care with a 'personhood lens'

In an attempt to address the psychological, social and neurological factors experienced by people with dementia, Kitwood (1997: 8) defined 'personhood' as 'the standing or status that is bestowed upon one human being, by others, in the context of relationship and social being'. Kitwood's definition, although limited in its recognition of the unique contribution of each person with dementia in a social context and thus confusing and contradictory (Macdonald 2018), focused attention on the importance of person-centred care. This focus, in turn, led to insight into the essential aspect of personhood – understanding and contextualising the reactions and perceptions of people with dementia, and enabling an approach to care that can keep those with dementia socially engaged.

Building on Kitwood's work, O'Connor and colleagues (2007) proposed an interdisciplinary, multi-perspective research framework focused on documenting the self-reported experiences of people with dementia in order to gain insight into the impact of these experiences on sense of self, identity and social contexts, particularly as the dementia progressed. Although definitions of person-centred and socially-engaged care continue to vary (e.g. Buron 2008; Hammer 2012; Smebye and Kirkevold 2013; Higgs and Gilleard 2016; Braddock 2017; Mascolo and Raeff 2017), understanding what it means to be a socially-engaged and valued person, despite a diagnosis of dementia, is especially relevant for those who provide care, and who may have difficulty communicating with people in their care (Jootun and McGhee 2011; Milte *et al.* 2016; Allwood *et al.* 2017; Macdonald 2018). Those who provide care, whether professionally or in an unpaid capacity, need to consider dementia as a shared, social experience and build this perspective into the core component of their care (Macdonald 2018). In this way, socially-engaged care can become the framework under which person-centred care with a 'personhood lens' is provided.

This socially-engaged framework highlights the role of dignity and its relationship to autonomy, respect and quality of life in defining personhood in the context of socially-engaged dementia care. Enhancing the dignity of people with dementia is essential to effective care across all dementia stages (Örulv and Nikku 2007; Marventano *et al.* 2015; Nikmat *et al.* 2015; Johnston *et al.* 2016) and has been remarked upon by Shorten (2017), the current Leader of the Opposition in the Australian Parliament. Dignity is a complex concept (Brennan 2014) and its meaning may vary between individuals and situations (Pringle *et al.* 2015). Dignity can be viewed both as an 'inherent, and inviolable quality and value within every human being' (Tranvåg *et al.* 2016: 579) and as a personal quality which is 'contingent and contextual' (van Gennip *et al.* 2016: 492), reflecting how people see themselves and how others see them. Dignity is tied to the integrity of the mind and body, and involves autonomy, self-respect and social engagement – key components of personhood.

However, a diagnosis of dementia threatens dignity through challenging a person's sense of self, and through potential negative interactions and experiences with others (van Gennip *et al.* 2016; Macdonald 2018). Brennan (2014:

89) asserts that 'every person is both worthy *and* worthy of our concern;' thus, dementia care must be dignity-preserving throughout all stages of the condition if quality of life is to be optimised (Tranvåg *et al.* 2013, 2015, 2016).

Caregivers, whether family members or professionals, need to be supported in being aware that their actions can trigger both positive and negative reactions as their relationship with people with dementia is dynamic and ever-changing. Family caregivers often know more than professionals in this regard and their knowledge needs to be valued and shared (Macdonald 2018). Positive interpersonal relationships and close emotional bonds support and sustain personhood for people with dementia, maintaining a sense of self and autonomy through the sharing of ideas, opinions, needs and wants (Smebye and Kirkevold 2013; Mitchell and Agnelli 2015; van Gennip *et al.* 2016). However, caregivers can just as easily contribute to relationships that undermine personhood and dignity (Smebye and Kirkevold 2013; van Gennip *et al.* 2016; Tolhurst *et al.* 2017). Caregivers may do this unknowingly through failing to acknowledge tasks and decisions people with dementia are capable of carrying out, not respecting their wishes, not providing opportunities for reciprocity of care and concern, not understanding the nuances of touch and other forms of non-verbal communication, focusing on task-oriented care, rushing people with dementia through care routines, using infantile or condescending language and excluding people with dementia from daily social conversations when they are physically present (Smebye and Kirkevold 2013; Heggestad *et al.* 2015; van Gennip *et al.* 2016). Caregivers in residential aged care communities may be particularly vulnerable to these negative triggers due to the task- and medically-oriented care that is characteristic of facilities that have yet to adopt a person-centred, socially-engaged model of care.

In a meta-synthesis of findings from studies on dignity-preserving care in diverse international settings, Tranvåg and colleagues (2013) identified two foundational themes. The first theme advocated autonomy and integrity for persons with dementia through caregivers (a) having compassion, (b) confirming the person's worthiness and sense of self, and (c) creating a humane and purposeful environment. Key terms to facilitate autonomy and integrity in everyday life included knowledge, respect, empathy, insight, flexibility, time, trust, confidence, honesty, freedom (with security), social engagement and ability to converse in ways that facilitated choices and a sense of control. The second theme focused on balancing decision-making when a person's decision-making capacity was compromised. Caregiver skills in calm persuasion and cooperation were highlighted, particularly regarding routine daily activities such as personal care and administering medications. Subsequent studies by these investigators (2015, 2016) have reinforced the importance of social engagement, relational interactions and the value of life-history in dignity-preserving care leading to promising practices.

When people with dementia are valued as unique individuals, engaging them in social situations and understanding and appreciating their life history will help caregivers develop compassionate and dignity-preserving care. It is also important to recognise that caregivers need to be treated with respect and dignity. This dignity-oriented, person-centred approach incorporates biological, psychological and social domains in its focus on each person with dementia (Spector and Orrell 2010). All members of the care team, including the person experiencing dementia-related life changes, work together to ensure dignity and respect are preserved, culturally appropriate and evidence-based care is provided, an ongoing and socially-engaged sense of self with appropriate autonomy is sustained and optimal quality of life for each person with dementia is maintained (Spector and Orrell 2010; Zaleta and Carpenter 2010; World Health Organization 2012; Beerens *et al.* 2015; Marventano *et al.* 2015; Nikmat *et al.* 2015; Power 2015; Brännmark 2017). This approach is championed by the American Geriatrics Society (2016), the World Health Organization (WHO) in its revised model of health (2002, 2012), the worldwide Dignity in Care campaign (Guideline Adaptation Committee 2016), the Department of Health (2016), the National Institute for Health and Clinical Excellence (2006) and Indigenous and tribal people's health (Anderson *et al.* 2016). It is understood as essential to help people with dementia to live well (Power 2015).

## Incorporating a personhood lens in socially-engaged dementia care: building on the knowledge and skills of those with dementia and their caregivers

Ensuring a focus on dignity and the individual psychological and social needs of people with dementia can change the focus of care from *reactive management of behaviours* to *proactive preservation of personhood*. This focus should minimise the need for crisis management, forced care, restraints, psychotropic medications, including for depression and agitation, and exclusion from enjoyed activities as the condition changes over time (Cohen-Mansfield *et al.* 2015; Marventano *et al.* 2015; Eritz *et al.* 2016). This seemingly simple change may have a profound effect on reducing the stigma of dementia and addressing the implicit power imbalance between the person with dementia and those who provide care and support (Kilduff 2014). This includes family members and professional caregivers, as well as members of the broader community such as police officers, shop assistants, lawyers, bank tellers and bus drivers. All play important roles in facilitating the social connectedness of people with dementia.

The majority (70 per cent) of paid caregivers in Australia work in residential aged care and are personal care attendants (PCAs). A high proportion (67 per cent) of PCAs hold a Certificate III in Aged Care which is considered to be the standard Vocational Education and Training level qualification for this occupation (Mavromaras *et al.* 2017). The certificate course is generally completed over 12 months (two days per week) and includes an orientation to dementia and dementia care. However, numerous shorter and unregulated courses in aged and dementia care exist and residential aged care facilities may not require direct care staff (PCAs) to complete any formal training or education in dementia care prior to their employment (Stirling *et al.* 2010). Once employed, 80 per cent of staff are reported to have received work-related training (Mavromaras *et al.* 2017).

A substantial number of people are paid to provide home care and support to those living with dementia; 84 per cent are community care workers. While work-related training is provided, the need for further training in dementia care remains a priority (Mavromaras *et al.* 2017).

Medical doctors, nurses and allied health professionals also provide care to those with dementia. Their approach is guided by the World Health Organization's revised biopsychosocial model, moving away from the traditional focus on a disabling medical condition to a focus on promoting health and wellbeing. However, as Macdonald (2018) suggests, this approach may inadvertently remain more 'biomedical' with less emphasis placed on the social, relational contexts in which those with dementia and their caregivers live and need to function.

A key element in dementia care is the support and care provided by unpaid or informal caregivers, whether such care is temporary or full-time. The burden of care can become overwhelming and increase the vulnerability of these informal caregivers to emotional distress and chronic disease, including dementia (Kraijo *et al.* 2015; Bottiggi Dassel *et al.* 2017). In order for informal caregivers to cope with the demands of care and sustain their own care, they need to be considered as integral members of any care team. Their knowledge of and insight into, the social and relational contexts that frame daily function, behaviours and effective care is essential information for all team members. Reciprocally, professional team members need to share their knowledge of the trajectory of dementia and evidence-based approaches to care, and work with informal caregivers to reduce the tensions frequently associated with balancing caregiving activities at home, social activities and paid work.

Despite existing educational and training programmes, awareness of the importance of team-based approaches, the availability of massive open online courses about dementia (Goldberg *et al.* 2015; Goldberg and Crocombe 2017) and an increased focus on dementia care by government and industry, dementia literacy and understanding of the need for socially-engaged care remain limited, particularly for those who provide direct care (Stirling *et al.* 2010; Andrews *et al.* 2017). Thus, socially-engaged and person-centred care through a 'personhood lens' remains elusive.

## The online bachelor of dementia care

To address this knowledge gap, the Wicking Dementia Research and Education Centre at the University of Tasmania has developed a fully online Bachelor of Dementia Care (BDC) degree. The 24-unit, three-year programme is centred on the WHO's biopsychosocial model of health and wellbeing. Rather than focusing on a disease, the WHO approach now incorporates biological, psychological and social domains in its focus on the *person* with the disease (Spector and Orell 2010). The BDC programme is organised into two vertical and integrated steams: 'Understanding Dementia' – the neuroscience of dementia, and 'Models of Healthcare' – the translation of current evidence into effective care. Units are taught by an experienced interdisciplinary team of neuroscientists, psychologists, nurses, pharmacists and allied health professionals to increase students' understanding of the dementia-related changes that occur in the brain, the signs and symptoms that result and the need for effective, multi-dimensional person-centred care to facilitate the social engagement of people with dementia. Early (Year 1) units such as *Introduction to Dementia Services* (CAD103) and *Principles of Supportive Care for People with Dementia* (CAD104) set the stage for continued learning about social and relational issues in dementia care, addressing concepts of discrimination, ageism, social exclusion and marginalisation, and the importance of dementia-friendly and community-wide approaches to care.

The programme is open to anyone seeking to learn more about dementia but is specifically designed to attract and support people who are providing direct care, whether that care is paid or unpaid, and at home, in the community or in a residential aged care setting. Students can study full- or part-time and there are two early completion points: a Diploma after completing eight units and an Associate Degree after completing 16 units. Currently, there are approximately 1200 enrolled students; 80 per cent are involved in care provision, whether through medicine, rehabilitative therapy, nursing – both in management and support roles, or personal (paid and unpaid) care. The remaining 20 per cent of students are those in other university programmes who are completing programme units as study electives, e.g. the Bachelor of Medicine, Bachelor of Nursing, Bachelor of Paramedic Practice and Bachelor of Social Work.

Programme material is deliberately scaffolded to reinforce and build on previously completed content. In the Year 1 unit, *Principles of Supportive Care for People with Dementia*, which is the focus of this chapter, material emphasises person-centred and dignity-preserving care across the trajectory of dementia. Material is made authentic through a 'personhood lens' with an interwoven story of a couple, Irene and David, and their experiences about living with dementia. Students interact with Irene and David through recorded interviews, documented experiences and a video conference. Through this real-life study, students learn to value the life history, environment, experiences and strengths of these two people, as well as the difficulties they encounter as David's dementia progresses.

Throughout the unit students are reminded that people living with a diagnosis of dementia are always seen as people, regardless of their capacity or mental state, and that their human rights and status are not diminished by their increasing cognitive, functional and behavioural impairments. Students are asked to reflect on the nature of their own attitudes towards people with dementia in the context of what they are learning about stigma and discrimination. Through online discussions, tutorials and guided reflective assignments, students are provided with opportunities to learn how a person-centred approach to care recognises and values each individual's personhood and social contexts. Students learn how to support this approach and educate others about its importance. Most importantly, students learn how to facilitate, appreciate and act on the expressions, verbal and non-verbal, people with dementia contribute about their experiences in their ongoing dementia journey.

## Insights from students as they applied their learning

A cohort of 346 students recently completed CAD104: *Principles of Supportive Care for People with Dementia*. The majority of these students worked directly (nurses, PCAs, family caregivers, allied health professionals, leisure and lifestyle coordinators, spiritual advisors) or indirectly (cooks, nutritional consultants, programme administrators) with people with dementia. At the end of the unit, students were asked to post a 300-word reflective commentary addressing one or more of the following areas: Which material had particular significance for them and why? What areas would they like to learn more about and why? Had they gained reassurance that their approach to care is supportive of people with dementia and those who care for them? Why or why not? Had they changed aspects of their approach or thinking to be more supportive of people with dementia and those who care for them? Why or why not? How had they helped to educate others about supportive approaches to care? and What were their impressions of the care experienced by the couple?

Students' reflections were de-identified and collated into a Microsoft Excel document for thematic analysis. Structural topic modelling with the R software package 'stm' (Roberts *et al.* 2014; R Core Team 2016) identified shared insights. These insights are illustrated in the following section and show the students' developing awareness of (i) the importance of person-centred care, (ii) how this is best achieved through a personhood lens to understand what a person with dementia may be experiencing and trying to communicate, and (iii) how others in the community can be enlightened about this approach. Students' comments indicated their willingness to *reframe* how they interpreted and responded to the behaviour of people with dementia.

## Understanding person-centred care

Students were awakened to understanding the importance of focusing on 'human-ness' first, and then the disease:

> The content of this course has really established my understanding that every person is a person first and foremost ...we remain that person and the disease process is simply a component of our life journey. A diagnosis of dementia should not be the end to a person living their life to the full, but rather the continuation of that life with recognition that additional support is likely to be needed into the future to continue that quality of life.
>
> [My] previous education in dementia has been heavily pathology-based and because of this I found myself unknowingly viewing dementia through

a biomedical lens. This unit actually shifted my view to the biopsychosocial model to incorporate the additional factors that accompany pathology on the dementia journey and focus on the person, the carers and staff.

They were awakened to the realisation that basic care was not the same as person-centred care:

> Person-centred care ... is far more important than just tending to basic care requirements. It shows the person with dementia that you care, respect and appreciate their participation and inclusion in all matters.
>
> Before this subject I was just going through the motions. I am a hospital trained registered nurse and have been working in aged care for many years looking at dementia care from a medical task-orientated aspect. I realise now how misinformed this has been – caring for the residents for our benefit, not wanting to getting to know them as 'real people.' Our routines were centred on what suited the staff.

Their awakening deepened to understanding how their care needed to, and could change:

> I have found myself acknowledging and spending more time with residents in terms of communication, rather than being focused on completing a task.
>
> I've grown old with the residents, been with them so much that they have ceased to be individuals to me but a group of people that require caring for. That is why learning about 'personhood' struck a chord with me, made me realise how much I disrespect my residents by not giving them their individuality ... I finally understood.

As these awakenings occurred, some students struggled with how to reframe their experiences in the language they used, particularly in changing to consider 'patients' as 'people' across care settings. Contradictions in their writing illustrated this struggle, as evident in the following reflection:

> I have found it interesting to realise how offensive it is to be called by a term of endearment. I am terrible with names. It can be hard to know which patient is which as patients change. I only work part-time and I do a reasonable amount of night duty, so I don't get to match names to faces all the time... I'm not convinced that patients should wear a name tag. I think there is definitely a case for people in aged care, I've done agency shifts and struggled with administering medications... but it's their own home and who wears a name tag in their own home? I'm not sure what the answer is.

Awakening to understanding the importance of a whole-of-system approach where the underlying concepts of person-centred care are valued in practise was a further shared insight, and is illustrated below:

As health professionals we hear the words 'person-centred care' but I now realise that very few people actually understand what is meant by person-centred care. I would love to see person-centred care being incorporated into one of the standards against which organisations are accredited. Particularly in hospitals where we talk a lot about person-centred care but the focus is essentially a medical approach. We talk about the illness rather than the person.

## Through a 'personhood lens'

Learning to view dementia through a lens that focused on what the condition might mean for those affected by it, helped students understand how knowing the person with dementia increased the chance of preserving dignity and optimising quality of life. Shared insights in students' comments reflected a change in attitude, behaviour and compassion and showed how they were open to new perspectives.

> I changed the moment I watched the video of Irene and David. Seeing them describe their journey made everything that they are going through real for me. I realized that David is the same as the residents that I care for at my work and Irene represents the families I deal with every day.
>
> Previously, I used to focus too much on the biomedical aspect of care … Now, I view my care recipients more holistically and it has opened my eyes to change my perception on things … this is not acute care. It is their home. And being such, care planning should be geared towards long term care and overall quality of life.

Students' comments documented how they valued and were challenged by their new learning about effective care and support, and most importantly, how they now saw people with dementia as people to be respected and considered, rather than as tasks to be completed.

> I thought I had to work within a biomedical model as I am dealing continuously with medications … I am now acutely aware of the importance of a resident's life story and social history … and have changed the way I interact.
>
> With a more complete understanding of the perceptions, existing abilities and requirements of people with dementia, I feel far more confident in providing care that is tailored to the client.

They shared insights addressed at recognising abilities, maintaining dignity and optimising quality of life in socially-engaged and person-centred care:

> My current approach is now grounded on peoples' abilities instead of their limitations. I see people with dementia as…not different to others and that

they have feelings and needs that should be supported. I am convinced that now I have the potential, right, and responsibility to change peoples' lives to be more meaningful through providing supportive services that inspire hope and confidence.

If we, as healthcare workers, can use a person-centred care approach to assist improvement in quality of life by understanding individuals' wants and needs, then perhaps people with dementia may feel more comfortable as they progress through the stages of the disease.

I understand more about why and how we undermine the personhood of someone with dementia, as well as participating, unwittingly or not, in their isolation, disenfranchisement and dehumanisation, in our fear and need to control.

I will be more communicative with the carers and try to gain a real understanding into what the person with dementia was like, what they enjoy, and hopefully incorporate this successfully into care.

[A person with dementia] is identified as an entire being. In other words, someone with a past and a history who [needs to be] afforded respect and dignity throughout their life.

## Recognising the need to educate others

Students developed more confidence in approaching staff and managers in their workplaces to reframe their role in shaping the care delivered and the attitudes of future health professionals:

I can now understand the signs of ill-being and how person-centred care can improve a person's quality of life. I can now more clearly recognise, label and explain care that is not person-centred. I am using this knowledge to improve the understanding of better practices of care with my fellow colleagues and hopefully the residents we provide care for will benefit.

I had never heard of person-centred care before, and yet I have fully bought into the principles behind it. It made me reflect long and hard about the way we treat our residents on the ward where I work, so much so, I asked my line manager if I could present the concept of person-centred care to the staff.

By modelling the practice of person-centred care I can support the person living with dementia and increase wellbeing.

I would like to be able to explain it [this model of care] to others…Currently I feel that there is no guiding principle in the work that I do with people in residential aged care facilities; treatment is on an as needs basis. It would be good to be more driven by the needs of the clients rather than the requests of the staff…we sometimes do not take a holistic view of the client.

I have shared much of what I have learned this semester with the [first year nursing] students with whom I work as well as the staff employed within the [residential aged care] facility. The students have unanimously stated that they have an entirely new appreciation for the value of aged care and specifically caring for people with dementia. I am hopeful that with time, each of these emerging nurses will also share that knowledge and experience and ultimately change the way [we] care for people with dementia in both the acute and long-term care settings.

## Implications

The analysis of students' reflections at the end of a 13-week, first year unit focused on the concept of person-centred care, identified important insights, growth in knowledge and students' desire to translate this new knowledge into more effective care. Asked to consider the perspective of the person with dementia, and to respect and support individual personhood, dignity and rights, students' reflections showed their increasing awareness that each person with dementia must be considered as a person first, engaged in meaningful social and relational contexts, and understood as having a medical condition second. Further, that dignity and a sense of self need to be at the heart of person-centred care in daily life and how the preservation of personhood is integral to effective care. Of equal importance, students valued the knowledge and perspective of those who provide care, particularly informal caregivers, and how caregivers' knowledge and perspective need to be incorporated for effective and authentic care.

This emerging awareness validated the intent of the CAD104 unit. The challenge for teaching staff, as well as the students, is to ensure that the presentation and discussion of socially-engaged, relationship-based and person-centred care through a 'personhood lens' is highlighted and deepened in the Models of Healthcare units that follow in Years 2 and 3 of the Bachelor of Dementia Care programme. Further, that students are supported when they are confronted by work-place challenges in planning socially-engaged care to meet individual needs and preferences, and how such planning needs to be guided by the people at the centre of this care.

## Conclusion

Dementia is recognised as a global public health issue and the importance of person-centred, socially-engaged care is widely accepted. However, dementia literacy remains limited, particularly for people who provide direct care. Socially-engaged, person-centred care, planned and delivered through a 'personhood lens', remains elusive. Guided online learning about dementia and evidence-based care, as illustrated in this chapter, can be one effective strategy in the challenge to educate caregivers and equip them with the confidence to implement care that supports each individual's personhood, educates others and contributes to quality of social life across the lifespan to benefit all who are living with dementia.

To live life well, people with dementia must be understood as citizens in society, regardless of the setting in which they receive support and care. This understanding entails taking the time to get to know what contributes to their uniqueness as people – their personhood and social value – and appreciating how their lifetime experiences, insights and needs are vital to shaping person-centred care as dementia progresses. This 'personhood lens' enables care that is based on dignity, respect and appropriate autonomy; care that is compassionate and culturally safe; care that enhances quality of life and social engagement; and care that decreases vulnerability to stigma and discrimination. Dementia education and training programmes need to reflect this approach to care.

## Note

1 The development of this paper was supported with funding from the JO and JR Wicking Trust (Equity Trustees). Ethics approval for this work was obtained from the Tasmanian Social Sciences Human Research Ethics Committee (HREC #H13822).

## References

Allwood, R., A. Pilnick, R. O'Brien, S. Goldberg, R. Harwood, S. Beeke, 2017, Should I stay or should I go? How healthcare professionals' close encounters with people with dementia in the acute hospital setting, *Social Science and Medicine*, 191: 212–225.

American Geriatrics Society, 2016, Person-centered care: A definition and essential elements, *Journal of the American Geriatrics Society*, 64: 15–18.

Anderson, I., B. Robson, M. Connolly, F. Al-Yaman, E. Bjertness, A. King, M. Tynan, R. Madden, A. Bang, C.E.A. Coimbra, M.A. Pesantes, H. Amigo, S. Andronov, B. Armien, D.A. Obando, P. Axelsson, Z.S. Bhatti, Z.A. Bhutta, P. Bjerregaard, M.B. Bjertness, R. Briceno-Leon, A.R. Broderstad, P. Bustos, V. Chongsuvivatwong, J. Chu, J. Gouda, R. Harikumar, T.T. Htay, A.S. Htet, C. Izugbara, M. Kamaka, M. King, M.R. Kodavanti, M. Lara, A. Laxmaiah, C. Lema, A.M.L. Taborda, T. Liabsuetrakul, A. Lobanov, M. Melhus, I. Meshram, J.J. Miranda, T.T. Mu, B. Nagalla, A. Nimmathota, A.I. Popov, A.M.P. Poveda, F. Ram, H. Reich, R.V. Santos, A.A. Sein, C. Shekhar, L.Y. Sherpa, P. Skold, S. Tano, A. Tanywe, C. Ugwu, F. Ugwu, P. Vapattanawong, X. Wan, J.R. Welch, G. Yang, Z. Yang, L. Yap, 2016, Indigenous and tribal people's health, (The Lancet-Lowitja Institute Global Collaboration), A population study, *The Lancet*, 388: 131–157.

Andrews, S., F. McInerney, C. Toye, C.A. Parkinson, A. Robinson, 2017, Knowledge of dementia: Do family members understand dementia as a terminal condition?, *Dementia*, 16(5): 556–575.

Beerens, H.C., S.M.G. Zwakhalen, H. Verbeek, D. Ruwaard, A.W. Ambergen, H. Leino-Kilpi, A. Stephan, A. Zabalegui, M. Soto, K. Saks, C. Bökberg, C.L. Sutcliffe, J.P.H. Hamers, on behalf of the RightTimePlaceCare Consortium, 2015, Change in quality of life of people with dementia recently admitted to long-term care facilities, *Journal of Advanced Nursing*, 71(6): 1435–1446.

Bottiggi Dassel, K., D.C. Carr, P. Vitaliano, 2017, Does caring for a spouse with dementia accelerate cognitive decline?: Findings from the health and retirement study, *The Gerontologist*, 57(2): 319–328.

Braddock, M., 2017, Should we treat vegetative and minimally conscious patients as persons?, *Neuroethics*, 10: 267–280.

Brännmark, J., 2017, Patients as rights holders, *Hastings Center Report*, July-August, 32–39.

Brennan, F., 2014, Dignity: A unifying concept for palliative care and human rights, *Progress in Palliative Care*, 22(2): 88–96.

Buron, B., 2008, Levels of personhood: A model for dementia care, *Geriatric Nursing*, 29(5): 324–332.

Cohen-Mansfield, J., M. Dakheel-Ali, M. Marx, K. Thein, N. Regier, 2015, Which unmet needs contribute to behavior problems in persons with advanced dementia?, *Psychiatry Research*, 228: 59–64.

Department of Health., 2016, *Charter of Care Recipients' Rights and Responsibilities – Residential Care*, https://agedcare.health.gov.au/publications-and-articles/guides-advice-and-policies/charter-of-care-recipients-rights-and-responsibilities-residential-care.

Eritz, H., T. Hadjistavropoulos, J. Williams, K. Kroeker, R.R. Martin, L.M. Lix, P. Hunter, 2016, A life history intervention for individuals with dementia: A randomised controlled trial examining nursing staff empathy, perceived patient personhood and aggressive behaviours, *Ageing and Society*, 36: 2061–2089.

Goldberg, L.R., L.A. Crocombe, 2017, Advances in medical education and practice: Role of Massive Open Online Courses, *Advances in Medical Education and Practice*, 8: 603–609.

Goldberg, L.R., E. Bell, C. King, C. O'Mara, F. McInerney, A. Robinson, J. Vickers, 2015, Relationship between participants' level of education and engagement in their completion of the Understanding Dementia Massive Open Online Course, *BMC Medical Education, Approaches to Teaching and Learning*, 15: 60.

Guideline Adaptation Committee., 2016, *Clinical Practice Guidelines and Principles of Care for People with Dementia*, Sydney: Guideline Adaptation Committee.

Hammer, J., 2012, Absolute personhood in those with dementia, *Georgetown University Journal of Health Sciences*, 6(2).

Heggestad, A.K.T., P. Nortvedt, Å Slettebø, 2015, Dignity and care for people with dementia living in nursing homes, *Dementia*, 14(6): 825–841.

Higgs, P., C. Gilleard, 2016, Interrogating personhood and dementia, *Aging and Mental Health*, 20(8): 773–780.

Johnston, B., S. Lawton, C. McCaw, *et al.*, 2016, Living well with dementia: Enhancing dignity and quality of life, using a novel intervention, Dignity Therapy, *International Journal of Older People Nursing*, 11: 107–120.

Jootun, D., G. McGhee, 2011, Effective communication with people who have dementia, *Nursing Standard*, 25(25): 40–46.

Kilduff, A., 2014, Dementia and stigma: A review of the literature on the reality of living with dementia, *Mental Health Nursing*, 34(5): 7–11.

Kitwood, T., 1997, *Dementia Reconsidered: The Person Comes First*, Berkshire, UK: Open University Press.

Kraijo, H., J. van Exel, W. Brouwer, 2015, The perseverance time of informal carers for people with dementia: Results of a two-year longitudinal follow-up study, *BMC Nursing*, 14: 56.

Macdonald, G., 2018, Death in life or life in death?: Dementia's ontological challenge, *Death Studies*, 42(5), 290–297.

Marventano, S., M-E. Prieto-Flores, B. Sanz-Barbero, S. Martin-Garcia, G. Fernandez-Mayoralas, F. Rojo-Perez, P. Martinez-Martin, M.J. Forjaz, on behalf of Spanish research group on quality of life and ageing, 2015, Quality of life in older people with dementia: A multilevel study of individual attributes and residential care center characteristics, *Geriatric and Gerontological International*, 15: 104–110.

Mascalo, M., C. Raeff, 2017, Understanding personhood: Can we get there from here?, *New Ideas in Psychology*, 44: 49–53.

Mavromaras, K., G. Knight, L. Isherwood, A. Crettenden, J. Flavel, T. Karmel, M. Moskos, M.L. Smith, H. Walton, Z. Wei, 2017, *The Aged Care Workforce, 2016*, Canberra, Australia: Australian Government Department of Health.

Milte, R., W. Shulver, M. Killington, C. Bradley, J. Ratcliffe, C. Crotty, 2016, Quality in residential care from the perspective of people living with dementia: The importance of personhood, *Archives of Gerontology and Geriatrics*, 63: 9–17.

Mitchell, G., J. Agnelli, 2015, Person-centred care for people with dementia: Kitwood reconsidered, *Nursing Standard*, 30(7): 46–50.

National Institute for Health and Clinical Excellence, 2006, *Dementia: Supporting People with Dementia and their Carers in Health and Social Care*, London: The Stationery Office.

Nikmat, A.W., G. Hawthorne, S.H. Al-Mashoor, 2015, The comparison of quality of life among people with mild dementia in nursing home and home care: A preliminary report, *Dementia*, 14(1): 114–125.

O'Connor, D., A. Phinney, A. Smith, J. Small, B. Purves, J. Perry, E. Drance, M. Donnelly, H. Chaudhury, L. Beattie, 2007, Personhood in dementia care, *Dementia*, 6(1): 121–142.

Örulv, L., N. Nikku, 2007, Dignity work in dementia care, *Dementia*, 6(4): 507–525.

Power, G.A., 2015, Well-being: A strengths-based approach to dementia, *Australian Journal of Dementia Care*, 4(2).

Prince, M., A. Wimo, M. Guerchet, G-C. Ali, Y-T. Wu, M. Prina, 2015, *World Alzheimer Report 2015: The Global Impact of Dementia: An Analysis of Prevalence, Incidence, Cost and Trends*, London: Alzheimer's Disease International (ADI).

Pringle, J., B. Johnston, D. Buchanan, 2015, Dignity and patient-centred care for people with palliative care needs in the acute hospital setting: A systematic review, *Palliative Medicine*, 29(8): 675–694.

R Core Team, 2016, *R: A Language and Environment for Statistical Computing*, Vienna, Austria: R Foundation for Statistical Computing.

Roberts, M.E., B.M. Stewart, D. Tingley, 2014, Stm: R package for structural topic models, *Journal of Statistical Software*, 59.

Shorten, B., 2017, *Tackling Dementia*, www.billshorten.com.au/tackling_dementia_our_generation_s_duty_sydney_tuesday_21_november_2017.

Slavin, M.J., H. Brodaty, P.S. Sachdev, 2013, Challenges of diagnosing dementia in the oldest old population, *Journal of Gerontology Series A: Biological Sciences and Medical Sciences*, 68(9): 1103–1111.

Smebye, K., M. Kirkevold, 2013, The influence of relationships on personhood in dementia care: A qualitative, hermeneutic study, *BMC Nursing*, 12(29): 1–13.

Spector, A., M. Orrell, 2010, Using a biopsychosocial model of dementia as a tool to guide clinical practice, *International Psychogeriatrics*, 22(6): 957–965.

Stirling, C.M., S. Andrews, T. Croft, A. Robinson, 2010, Measuring dementia carers' unmet need for services – An exploratory mixed method study, *BMC Health Services Research*, 10(1): 122.

Tolhurst, E., B. Weicht, P. Kingston, 2017, Narrative collisions, sociocultural pressures and dementia: The relational basis of personhood reconsidered, *Sociology of Health and Illness*, 39(2): 212–226.

Tranvåg, O., K.A. Petersen, D. Nåden, 2013, Dignity-preserving dementia care: A meta-synthesis, *Nursing Ethics*, 20(8): 861–880.

Tranvåg, O., K.A. Petersen, D. Nåden, 2015, Relational interactions preserving dignity experience: Perceptions of persons living with dementia, *Nursing Ethics*, 22(5): 577–593.

Tranvåg, O., K.A. Petersen, D. Nåden, 2016, Crucial dimensions constituting dignity experience in persons living with dementia, *Dementia*, 15(4): 578–595.

van Gennip, I.E., H.R.W. Pasman, M.G. Oosterveld-Vlug, D.L. Willems, B.D. Onwuteaka-Philipsen, 2016, How dementia affects personal dignity: A qualitative study on the perspective of individuals with mild to moderate dementia, *Journals of Gerontology Series B: Social Sciences*, 71(3): 491–501.

World Health Organization, 2002, *Towards a Common Language for Functioning, Disability and Health*, Geneva, Switzerland: World Health Organization.

World Health Organization, 2012, *Dementia: A Public Health Priority*, Geneva, Switzerland: World Health Organization.

Zaleta, A.K., B.D. Carpenter, 2010, Patient-centered communication during the disclosure of a dementia diagnosis, *American Journal of Alzheimers Disease and Other Dementias*, 25(6): 513–520.

# 10  Emotional labour, person-centred care and problem solving in regulating dementia care

*Ashley Carr and Simon Biggs*

## Introduction

This chapter focuses on the interactions between care workers and people with dementia within the context of residential care. Linking the person-centred care and emotional labour literatures reveals the multiple, often competing, demands care workers face in their daily work, particularly the various care needs of residents and the emotional work involved in dementia care. We use regulation as a lens to explore the different strategies care workers deploy to manage and balance these demands. One of these strategies involves using regulatory rules to guard against uncertainty and emotional engagement, in the process eclipsing the intent of regulation and the relational qualities of care. An alternative, more creative strategy is to approach dementia and dementia care as a puzzle that needs unravelling and piecing together. In this approach, care workers combine empathy, professional distancing and problem-solving to balance, in more productive ways, daily care, emotional work and the regulatory rules intended to govern their conduct. The findings provide new insights into the theory and practice of dementia care, particularly in the context of regulation.

Regulation is one of the ways governments manage care at a distance and manage a mixed economy of care. Through a regulatory framework, administered by the Australian Government, relevant departments and various regulatory agencies and by stipulating the rules, care standards and accountabilities under which care providers operate, regulations shape a social environment for the conduct of care. This is important for maintaining care standards, protecting the vulnerable and controlling care conduct, all central concerns in the governance of residential aged care. However, while largely understood as objective, targeted and instrumental (Haines 2011), regulation can have unintended consequences, and may be interpreted differently depending on the care setting.

Care provider organisations and their workers respond to standardised regulations in different ways. Care workers in particular strategise their conduct in light of competing demands, including regulatory control, the different and changing needs of individual care recipients and the emotions involved in their work. These demands are particularly important in the context of residential care for people living with dementia.

Engaging key elements of the person-centred care (patient oriented) and emotional labour (care professional oriented) literatures, which can seem as if they are contradictory, provides the basis for exploring the strategies that care workers deploy in their daily work. These strategies reveal how regulation, care and emotional labour might be integrated. Our findings suggest, on the one hand, that regulation can be used to help care workers manage the uncertainties of daily care and the complex emotions involved, and on the other, can also be used to provide a broad framework within which flexible and creative approaches to care are possible.

## Aged care regulation in Australia

The Australian Government (2014: 3, 62) describes regulation as 'any rule endorsed by government where there is an expectation of compliance', which 'includes legislation, regulations, quasi-regulations and any other aspect of regulator behaviour which can influence or compel specific behaviour by business, community organisations or individuals'; and as a 'key tool for achieving ... the policy objectives of governments' (Australian National Audit Office 2014: 3). Key policy and regulatory objectives of aged care are contained within the *Aged Care Act 1997* and related *Principles*, followed by other relevant Commonwealth and State regulations. The *Act* and relevant *Principles* specify what residents are entitled to receive, a Charter of Residents' Rights and Responsibilities, a set of national quality care standards and the means by which the standards are monitored and enforced (*Quality Principles 2014* made under the *Aged Care Act 1997*; Australian Government Department of Health 2016).

Policy reform has been incorporated within the broad regulatory framework and through amendments to the *Act*. For instance, over time dementia care has become a central part of the aged care system, achieved through service developments, specific funding arrangements and regulation. More recently new regulatory arrangements have been introduced as part of making aged care more consumer-driven. Measures, such as the requirement for organisations to implement personalised budgets for their clients and facilitate greater degrees of choice around care provision and service, have been introduced as part of a consumer-directed care (CDC) model (Australian Government Department of Health 2016). To date, these developments have not yet influenced residential care to the same degree as home and community care. As one government-contracted report suggests, numerous challenges exist in the implementation of CDC in residential care, including: the prevailing culture(s) of residential care, confusion around choice-making with respect to people living with dementia, and importantly, the perception of competing priorities in residential care settings, namely, between regulatory compliance and user-choice (KPMG 2014).

While recent reforms around increasing choice have been introduced in tandem with raising the contribution care users make towards financing their own care, aged care remains primarily government funded. Most of these funds ($11.4 billion of $16.2 billion, or two-thirds spent annually) are allocated to residential care services (Australian Government Department of Health 2016). This funding supports about 1000 approved residential care providers, comprising a mix of not-for-profit, for-profit and government organisations and agencies, who together operate nearly 2700 residential care facilities (not-for-profit religious, charitable and community organisations currently operate about 56 per cent of all residential care places, whereas for-profit and government operate about 39 per cent and 4.5 per cent, respectively). Just over half of all residential care facilities provide care to over 60 people and 80 per cent of these facilities are operated by a larger provider group (Australian Government Department of Health 2016).

In June 2016, residential care services provided care to approximately 175,000 residents, half of whom had a diagnosis of dementia (Australian Government Department of Health 2016). Their care is regulated through a national accreditation system, which covers four standards: (1) Management systems, staffing and organisational development, (2) Health and personal care, (3) Resident lifestyle and (4) Physical environment and safe systems (*Quality Care Principles 2014* made under the *Aged Care Act 1997*). The principle of 'continuous improvement' and 'compliance with all relevant legislation, regulatory requirements, professional standards, and guidelines', including State-based regulations, are contained within each standard (*Quality Care Principles 2014* made under the *Aged Care Act 1997*). The performance of care providers against the standards is monitored and enforced by the semi-independent Australian Aged Care Quality Agency and the relevant government department. The financing of care is regulated by the Aged Care Financing Authority, which conducts regular audits to monitor the funding claimed by providers on behalf of care recipients. Compliance with other relevant regulations, including food safety, fire safety, building design and workplace safety, is monitored by another set of regulatory agencies, usually state-based, thus adding another layer of regulation, audit and compliance.

If government statute consists of 'hard regulation', then its implementation in local care and organisational settings generates a layer of soft regulation. Soft forms interpret regulation in particular contexts, making it intelligible to practitioners. According to Freiberg (2010) 'soft' forms of law and regulation occupy 'a very large part of the regulatory terrain as is it experienced by most regulatees', and can include 'regulatory guides, rules or codes of conduct...declarations of policy and practice, management plans...interpretative guides or decisions'.

Provider organisations occupy a middle-ground in the governance of care, between governmental and regulatory authorities on the one hand, and the conduct and practise of care on the other. Through the development of 'soft regulation', namely, organisational policies, processes and other forms of guidance, which care workers are expected to follow, they translate hard regulations into daily practice. This process suggests an interpretive space with opportunities for flexibility in care. It shows as well how standardised regulatory controls are adapted to particular care settings, and critically, how multiple frames of reference are combined, and at times, compete, in formal care.

Pols (2004) has called these different frames of reference 'modes of ordering' discourses 'on a ... smaller scale' and sees them as useful for analysing 'everyday care practices'. As Mol *et al.* (2014) suggest, in care settings 'different ways of ordering reality have to be dealt with together', negotiated and tinkered with at the local level. This can create tensions. Armstrong (2017) demonstrates how this occurs between medical and social frames in residential care, leading to one priority overriding another. She suggests that, in the trade-off between the two, time is a critical issue, the lack of which 'often means a focus on essentials, and essentials are defined as medical'. These practices become taken for granted ways of doing things, from which beliefs and values are not just reflected but constituted (Hughes 2006). In daily care, this means that medical and clinical care may be prioritised over its relational and emotional elements.

## Person-centred care, emotional labour and regulation

The literature on dementia care has reflected two dominant discourses, person-centred care (centred ostensibly on the individual older person) and care as emotional labour (care workers) that have been used to frame research in this area. Both analyse and interrogate the strategies that care workers deploy in order to manage the tasks and emotional demands of their daily work. Influential arguments include Tom Kitwood's (1997) Person-Centred Care, which critiqued traditional care practices, emphasising increased empathic engagement and building caring relationships. Arlie Hochschild's (1983) work on emotional labour focuses on the burdens of emotional care work for care workers and the importance of building relationships. In contemporary literature on care, regulation and dementia, these two trends have existed in parallel rather than being connected or used together to capture the various dimensions that comprise aged and dementia care.

Person-centred care, in principle, 'values all people regardless of age and health status, is individualized, emphasizes the perspective of the person with dementia, and stresses the importance of relationships' (Brooker 2005: 11). It generally refers to the maintenance of personhood, as the 'standing or status that is bestowed upon one human being by others in the context of relationship and social being. It implies recognition, respect and trust' (Kitwood 1997: 8).

While proving difficult to detect, evaluate and measure (McCormack 2004), person-centred care has become a touchstone amongst care providers, most of whom declare commitment to the idea in principle and practice (Venturato *et al.* 2011). Perhaps the most important element of person-centred care is what Behuniak (2010) posits as one of Kitwood's central claims: while the disease robbed individuals of certain abilities, it was society that took away personhood; residential care was considered especially effective at undermining personhood (Kitwood and Bredin 1992).

The focus on inter-personal relations, has inspired various person-centred care models, such as the Burford Model, the Authentic Consciousness Framework and the Senses Framework (for a review of these models see McCormack 2004 and

Hunter *et al.* 2016). These models suggest different ways that the person-centred principles have been adapted to local settings, and crucially how dementia care practice has moved beyond focusing solely on the person to emphasise its relational and social dynamics. McCormack (2004) for instance, argues that person-centred dementia care comprises four aspects of the patient's experience: relationships, social being, environment and identity. Brooker (2007), under the 'VIPS' framework, highlights four elements of person-centredness: Values, Individualised approaches, the Perspective of the person receiving care and the Social environment. In these examples, person-centred care is achieved by balancing and integrating multiple components of care. In such an endeavour, the organisational setting and the support provided to direct care workers is considered to be of critical importance (McCormack 2003; Brooker 2007). However, evidence from the care workforce suggests that the organisational setting in which care is provided is not always conducive to person-centred care, and that care workers largely feel unsupported in their roles. A recent survey of the aged care workforce reports that personal care assistants in particular believe that they are not provided with sufficient training and the guidance needed to care for people with dementia, particularly at the inter-personal level (Mavromaras *et al.* 2017).

For these reasons, and more discussed below, person-centred care is taken for granted within aged care, and there has been little critique of the concept, particularly its application within policy and organisational settings. There is a general assumption that person-centred care improves wellbeing, particularly for people with dementia, with some linking the concept to the policy frame of CDC (see KPMG 2014), and suggesting widespread support for the practice amongst aged care providers (Venturato *et al.* 2011; KPMG 2014). What essentially unites the various models of person-centred care is attention to the person hidden behind cognitive decline. This involves, according to Herskovits (1995), acts of translation, whereby formal and informal carers assist people with dementia to express feelings that cannot be conveyed effectively.

Lawton (2000, cited in Davis 2004: 377) has argued that Kitwood offered an 'idea of unimpeachable personhood, which sanitises the dying process'. This places formal and informal carers in a tenuous position. If personhood cannot be maintained, as Davis (2004) argues, carers can be seen as complicit in its 'dissolution'. For example, carers might also be required to assume a more constructive role, curating expressions of self-identity to 'reproduce and reconfirm' personhood (Crichton and Koch 2007; Buse and Twigg 2016). Failure to succeed in this task can likewise compound the emotional demands of care work. Informal and formal care workers are thus charged with responsibilities that are emotionally demanding and potentially set them up to fail. As such, the emotional work involved in dementia care needs to be seen as an essential component of person-centredness, and the importance of inter-personal relationships in care settings and the relational focus of dementia care work that has begun to emerge needs to be acknowledged.

The term 'emotional labour' was first considered by Hochschild (1983: 7) and defined as 'the management of feeling to create a publicly observable facial and bodily display', requiring, 'one to induce or suppress feelings in order to sustain the outward countenance that produces the proper state of mind in others – in this case, the sense of being cared for in a convivial and safe place'. While originally developed in the context of the work done by flight attendants, emotional labour has since been applied in various other settings, including aged and dementia care. Fine (2015), for example, identifies emotional labour as an important consideration in defining cultures of aged care, specifically what Hochschild (2003) referred to as the 'cold modern' approach of institutionalised care, which lacked true feelings of warmth and sympathy. Lopez (2006) argues, in the context of nursing home care for people with dementia, that emotional labour acts as a coercive force by which employers prescribe certain feeling rules on workers. He proposes instead the notion of 'organized emotional care', defined as 'organizational attempts to create hospitable conditions for the development of caring relationships', and arguably a more genuine approach towards 'caring about' and 'caring for' (Tronto 1994) people with dementia. When adopted as part of an organisational strategy for managing care, 'organized emotional care' can be achieved by the use of soft regulations – 'rules, procedures, and record-keeping'– to encourage 'relationship building and emotional honesty' in staff-resident interactions (Lopez 2006: 137).

Bailey and colleagues (2015) observed that emotional contact and empathy are difficult for formal care workers to establish in dementia care settings; feelings are often ambivalent, ambiguous and the values and meanings of care are not always shared between workers and residents. 'The environment of the dementia ward offers ... a particularly ambiguous set of feeling rules', that, in combination with the feelings of multiple parties, including co-workers, families and residents, creates an uncertain emotional environment (Bailey *et al.* 2015: 252).

In order to navigate this uncertain emotional environment, along with the stresses associated with feeling overworked and short of time, care workers have been shown to rely heavily on routinised work and rule-following (see DeForge *et al.* 2011; Banerjee *et al.* 2015). Drawing on the work of Menzies Lyth (1988), whose study on nurse-patient relations in a London teaching hospital documented the different ways nurses cope with emotion engagement, Hoggett (2000: 57) argues: 'Routinisation provide workers with a way of not thinking or feeling too much...[as] a way of containing anxiety and other negative emotions aroused by working with the sick, the dying, the distressed...'. The need to respond to the nature of daily care work, and the strong and conflicted feelings that such work evokes, may prompt care workers to use routines and rule-following to guard against emotional contact with residents. Routinised work, particularly that predicated on paperwork and audit, becomes 'a simulacrum for real contact' (Hoggett 2000: 44). This approach contradicts the very characteristics that advocates of person-centred care, and later relational care, intended to correct (Kitwood 1997; Brooker 2004, 2007).

However, as Bailey and colleagues (2015) observed, routines do not have to be enacted in unfeeling or reductive ways, or leave no room for positive interaction. By balancing engagement with detachment, care routines can be enacted with empathy, enabling care workers to attend to the individual care and emotional needs of residents in creative ways. Nonetheless, tensions remain between the requirements of empathic person-centred care, the emotional labour involved and the dynamic of responding to regulatory environments.

Care work has emotional dimensions not always seen as a priority in dementia care policy and practice. Person-centred care in particular requires a level of emotional engagement that, when taken for granted or not acknowledged, creates particular challenges for the organisation and its workers. As the emotional labour literature indicates, care workers adopt and deploy various strategies to manage and contain the emotions involved in their work. Understanding how this occurs in the context of regulation provides an opportunity to reframe the analysis of formal dementia care and reconsider the strategies that care workers might adopt.

## The research: strategies adopted by direct care workers in dementia care

In what follows we draw on research interviews conducted with those working in residential care, specifically within not-for-profit facilities providing care to people with dementia. These interviews were conducted as part of a wider study on the role of regulation in aged and dementia care, which examined the effects of regulation at the system, organisational and practice-based levels. The interviews with direct care workers were part of an attempt to understand the role and effects of regulation in an organisational setting and in daily practice.

A total of 60 semi-structured, in-depth interviews were conducted with three distinct levels of organisation within three aged care provider organisations. The facility managers and care workers covered eight residential care facilities, with an average of five care workers from each facility (two of the care facilities were represented by one and two care workers, respectively). A total of 17 senior managers (SM), 13 facility managers (FM) and 30 direct care workers (CW) participated. Most of the participants were female – 13 of the 17 senior managers, all of the facility managers and 26 of the 30 care workers. The median age for senior managers was 48 years, for facility managers 49 years and for care workers 38 years. Senior managers held high-level management positions, often responsible for a particular area of care, including as part of this sample, quality and risk management, clinical care management, operational management (residential care), facility and property management, food and related services and marketing/communications. Facility managers were responsible for the day-to-day running and operations of a single facility, including the management of care staff, care provision on a day-to-day basis and accreditation. Care workers were responsible for daily care, including interacting with residents.

The interviews with all participants were conducted over the phone, lasted on average between 30 to 40 minutes and were conducted in confidence and independently of employers. The interview questions and information collected focused on the role of regulation in structuring daily routines. Care workers were asked to describe a typical day of work, and the role of regulation in structuring daily routines and care practice, specifically with respect to activities relating to food, morning and night routines and medication management. All participants were also given the opportunity to raise issues related to daily dementia care they thought significant and any area of regulation they experienced as important.

### *Regulating daily care*

In this section we outline the role of regulation in daily care work, focusing specifically on the care worker perspective to show how they respond to different forms of regulation. In direct care soft forms of regulation are designed at the more senior levels of organisation to make it 'as easy as possible for the care worker on the shop floor to know what their regulatory requirements are' (SM 3). This is done, according to senior managers, by incorporating regulatory compliance into daily routines and care procedures, with one in particular commenting on the benefits of having 'a group within the organisation that can filter changes in legislation and changes in standards' to the direct care level (SM 15).

Many care workers conveyed an experience of regulation in terms of the processes relating to workplace safety, food safety and medication management. One care worker described how formal laws and legislation became part of organisational processes:

> A newer care worker would have to have guidance ... if I was giving medication, for example, a lot of that would come with our policy, and that would give mention to the Therapeutic Goods Regulation [and] that part ... becomes almost irrelevant to the care worker. The policy becomes it.
>
> (CW 24)

Organisational policies and guidance not only included rules around daily care activities, such as assisting residents to get up in the morning, showering and food provision, but extended to conduct around resident-staff interactions.

Referring to organisational policies and procedures, and the direction provided by facility managers, a care worker stated: '[W]e're always told how we should treat our residents and how we should speak to our residents' (CW 2), with others reporting organisational rules around how residents should be woken in the morning, how they should be addressed and physical contact.

By detailing how care workers should interact and address residents, these forms of guidance worked to translate regulation, including the Charter of Residents' Rights with its principles of 'dignity and respect', into daily practice. As a senior manager suggested: 'the quality care principles and the user rights ... that's what we base our policies and procedures on' (SM 10), which in turn facilitated guidance around speaking and interacting with residents in a respectful manner, for example, discouraging the use of 'pet names' (CW 2) or unwanted physical contact (CW 4).

Critical in navigating regulation was the ability of care workers to determine which rules had to be followed to the letter and which permitted flexibility and discretion. As one care worker suggested, 'the rules and regulations concerning the individual, they have to bend because people are different ... But the proper regulations, as in food safety, OH&S [Occupational Health and Safety], medications and stuff ... they stay the same' (CW 17). For another, the 'really important stuff'–resident choice and interaction–was distinguished 'from the kind of rules that everyone has to follow' (CW 1).

At the individual and interactional levels flexibility in applying rules was required and was often compared with what care workers understood as the standardised or 'proper' rules designed primarily for safe practice. Thus, some workers accepted breaking or bending rules as a matter of course. '[Y]ou've got to break them sometimes for the comfort of the residents' (CW 15), states a care worker, referring to set bedtimes, while another suggests: 'we bend the rules a lot because it is dementia ... You have to otherwise we wouldn't be able to get our job done' (CW 23), with respect to allowing families to cook and bring food in for their loved ones.

As these quotes suggest, care workers often conflated 'hard' and 'soft' regulations, though were more likely to bend or break (or at least admit to bending or breaking) the guidance provided through organisational policies and procedures. Only a few care workers provided instances of not following the 'proper' procedures related to food safety, manual handling and medications.

Senior and facility management assisted care workers to negotiate multiple demands, including regulation, in a number of ways, including clear guidance around roles and regulatory requirements, ongoing support and training and counselling services. Most importantly, they could help provide an environment that was more relaxed, providing space for positive interactions. This could involve not insisting on the completion of tasks within unrealistic timeframes, staggering staff start times or supporting care workers in their interactions with regulators.

Overall, care workers expressed some ambivalence about the benefits of regulation, particularly, organisational policies and procedures. Daily dementia care was commonly reported as uncertain and unpredictable. '[Y]ou never know what you're in for', states a care worker, 'you never know ... how a person's going to respond ... So that affects what's going to happen each day' (CW 13). '[T]here's a lot of behaviours', states another, 'that can stop you from doing your job and fulfilling the task' (CW 23). And again: 'on any given day ... the routine can be thrown out of whack from the minute we walk in the door' (CW 21). Facility managers in particular were aware of the stress this could place on care workers. '[W]orking with people with really challenging behaviours all the time is very wearing for staff', stated a facility manager, 'it's very easy [for staff] to burn out' (FM 12). As such, most facility managers recognised the need to support staff, which for one was about using the 'carrot' rather than the 'stick', and monitoring their wellbeing (FM 11).

In the context of work that was 'stop-start' according to one care worker (CW 17), regulation was valued for the sense of order it provided. By defining roles and responsibilities, rules to guide practice and processes for reporting risk, it provided a level of certainty. 'The advantage is that everybody has to follow that thing ... if there is no rules and regulations, everything will get messed up' (CW 12), states a care worker, while another suggests: 'if you don't have the rules and regulations you have anarchy in the workplace' (CW 21). A number of care workers relied heavily on regulatory rules for their own protection: 'I always follow the rules because if we follow the rules it'll be alright ... Otherwise it's not good' (CW 8). Another saw strict adherence to rules as a form of protection against injury: 'I have to follow them, because if something happens it's my fault. I have to follow by the book', but continued, stating: 'It's quite sad really sometimes ... it's hard for me especially when they pass away, it's sad, you cry' (CW 5).

The gap between soft regulation and the practise of care, the need for care workers to identify where opportunities for flexibility arose and the value they placed on regulation, suggests that care organisations and their workers do not respond to regulation mechanically, but strategise their work in light of competing demands. To draw out further these observations we focus on two strategies arising from our data. The first positions regulatory rules as the chief aim of care, consequently side-lining emotional connection. The second presents a more creative approach to staff-resident interactions, combining empathic understanding with detachment in a problem-solving approach.

### Stresses in dementia care regulation: mis-attention or attending to regulatory rules, not people

One strategy for resolving the tension between person-centred care and the emotional demands of care work is the use of regulation as a guard against the various stresses and emotional strains of daily care work. However, in this approach, satisfying regulatory rules becomes the chief focus of care. It is reflected in rountinised behaviour, reporting practices, timetabling that prevents interaction and an overly prescriptive approach to soft rules and guidance. This was first and foremost conditioned around time demands. As one care worker states: 'it's very busy in the mornings ... you have to get everyone up and usually we're expected to shower all residents now'; suggesting as well that 'some people feel that they need to push themselves and get them up in the morning and pull them out of bed' (CW 1). Others suggested that management priorities determined the morning rush: 'we just sometimes feel pressure because you feel like it's a short staff ... [and] the management, they think that every morning we can do same routine' (CW 12). Time in particular, and the sense of being short-staffed, was the primary barrier to emotional engagement and connection in staff-resident interactions.

Many were well aware that routinised behaviour, particularly during the morning rush, prevented carer-resident interactions. As one care worker states: 'We got only two staff, two carers for 16 residents, we will be showering until 10 o'clock or 10:30 ... it's rush rush every time ... we don't have enough time ... to interact with the residents' (CW 7).

This was a constant source of frustration, as another reflects: 'we are rushed in the dementia wing. We're very rushed...That's the saddest part ... they [residents] really can do with some company' (CW 13). Another respondent stresses time and staffing, rather than procedures or rules: 'sometimes there isn't enough time to give to the client ... if the client does need their hand held for longer, the procedure doesn't stop you from doing that, time ... does' (CW 16).

Whilst time pressures prevented emotional connection with residents, so too could regulatory rules and related processes. Referring to the guidance provided by organisational policies around 'unwanted physical contact', a care worker claimed:

> I think we need rules and regulations for everyone's protection ... there's so many ... things these days about touching residents and how you handle them ... you can't just go up and give someone a hug ... I think a lot find that really difficult.
>
> (CW 4)

Here soft regulation, interpreted rigidly, appeared to prohibit personal contact, an aspect of care that was, according to this care worker, impossible to prevent.

Another care worker felt that tasks and accompanying rules took precedence over engagement:

> When we've finished all our ADLs [activities of daily living] and we've done everything we can with the residents, then there's a break time ... if there's generally free time I feel that I might want to spend some time with a resident, I'll go into their room and put on television, so then watch it together to spend five minutes together. But, I don't know if that was part of the rules or not, I didn't know if we always had to do care staff stuff or if we were allowed to actually watch television with the residents ... it mightn't look as professional if you're meant to be working.
>
> (CW 1)

And another:

> My duty is to look after residents fulltime and I have to assist them with any of their needs like showering, toileting, to maintain their privacy, dignity, everything, and helping them, assisting them with their meals ... in our free time we just do some activities to recognise something like the family members ... we just try then to recall their memory and do such activities.
>
> (CW 12)

In both quotes 'free time' occurs after the completion of tasks, and is where engaging with a resident most likely takes place. According to a facility manager, care workers desire to spend more time with residents, 'but ... can't because they have to do paperwork' (FM 12). The paperwork and documentation requirements generated via regulation protected care workers and facility managers on another level: from the stresses involved in being scrutinised by regulators. This was, articulated by a facility manager as follows:

> I don't think there is a requirement that we need to document in a resident's progress notes every day. However, we still ask our staff to do that because we're scared that if we don't and something happens the governing bodies will come and look at the file and go 'Well you're not providing any care because nothing's written there'.
>
> (FM 10)

'I can happily say', states a facility manager, referring to a recent visit from the Quality Agency, 'that we didn't have any non-compliances, thanks to me telling these guys [care staff] what they should and shouldn't be doing, and them adhering to the rules and regulations' (FM 1). When tied to performance, as measured by regulatory agencies, rules potentially become ends in themselves.

While overly focusing on rules and regulatory requirements might reduce the stress associated with being monitored, it could be seen as detrimental to staff autonomy and care. As a senior manager suggests:

> people working in aged care have stopped the challenge, have stopped believing they have any sort of autonomy. I think there is this culture of we are guided by these rules and if we put our toe over the line. I mean if you get sanctioned in aged care you lose your funding.
>
> (SM 8)

Staff-resident interactions could also suffer. A facility manager expresses this view, stating: 'the amount of work that's generated because we come under so many different legislations which then takes you away from focusing on the resident's living experience I guess and the care that you can provide' (FM 10). A senior manager reflects how, in the organisation of care seen through the guise of regulation, engagement is side-lined:

> You feel like you don't have any breathing space to be creative and be yourself ... I think it's one of the risks of services ending up being driven by the legislation rather than by the people they care for, because they're there so often that we feel like we've got to meet them. And it's easier to go, you know what, if I do this bit of paper over here and I have everyone signing it then I meet the piece of legislation, but there's not necessarily that reflection on what does that mean for staff time and contact with our residents and our people and that engagement that they should be giving in that space.
>
> (SM 13)

In contrast, some forms of reporting and monitoring could reduce emotional strain and enable connections with residents. Reporting issues up to supervisors, or into electronic risk management systems, transferred responsibility so that care workers could concentrate on day-to-day interactions with residents, and not take emotional baggage home with them. More importantly, a number of facilities had introduced more flexible approaches to care routines. Staggered staff starts, for example, were used to reduce the pressure to perform morning tasks within set timeframes, and arguably facilitated a more relaxed approach to the traditional morning rush.

Nonetheless, staffing levels, paperwork and documentation and task performance continued to be experienced as preventing emotional connection. The danger therefore, is that care workers give attention to the surfaces of regulatory compliance rather than the underlying intent of care. In this scenario, regulations are followed, with varying degrees of rigidity, as ends in themselves, rather than read as a means to facilitate and ensure good care or foster positive staff-resident interactions. Moreover, in the trade-off between task and engagement, time demands, staffing and regulatory requirements can take precedence.

### Dementia as a puzzle

We found one coping strategy which appeared to combine the demands for empathy while managing the emotional demands of care work. That was to see the changing behaviour of people with dementia as a puzzle to be unravelled and pieced together, leading to a problem-solving approach. This worked by combining the empathic principles of person-centred care with the professional distance required to manage emotional labour.

### Empathic understanding

In line with Kitwood's (1997) call to emphasise feeling and emotion, an assumed inability for people with dementia to reason (or more appropriately unconventional reasoning) paved the way for care workers and their managers to see feeling states as driving 'behaviour', though often explained as emotional responses to environmental triggers. Many workers coped with this imperative through empathy – trying to put themselves into the shoes of the other. This involved, amongst other factors, attending to the emotions of residents with dementia. '[I]t's all about emotions', stated a facility manager, so 'it's more about how they're feeling, so we've got to try to manage their feelings' (FM 12).

This, according to another required an empathic approach: 'I always say to staff this is their world. We go into their world, we don't expect them to come into our world' (FM 8). And, '[I]t's not like office work', states a care worker, 'you're dealing with people, you're dealing with their fears and emotions and their confusion' (CW 17).

Commenting on how they interacted and first approached care recipients one care worker states that it: 'Depends upon their behaviour, which mood they have, happy mood or sad mood' (CW 10). As such, care workers often worked towards reducing distress: 'A lot of our residents are in a stage where they know that they're not remembering, so they get anxious and that's when the staff really need to reassure them' (FM 12).

Significantly, the emphasis on emotion helped facilitate empathic understanding. As one care worker states:

> With dementia I mean you have to kind of project a lot of how you would feel comfortable in the situation, because a lot of them can't communicate, so you have to sort of do [the] thinking for them. So, you have to be generally a very considerate person.
>
> (CW 1)

Such empathy extended to a consideration of the feelings people with dementia might be experiencing, and the desires or intentions they might be struggling to communicate. One facility manager commented:

> The ones that are in the early stages of dementia ... they may phase in and out of their disease and think, 'what am I doing here? I've got to go home', and they're searching. They're wandering, they're looking for something ... it's very hard to comfort them.
>
> (FM 1)

Empathy was not just about knowing the person, but being aware of how they had changed. This could create some friction with families, who according to one facility, may not understand or accept such changes: 'Because it can't be seen and because it's not often understood by families who come in, there's a lot of walking the journey with them, explaining that this is a progressive debilitating disease that has side effects' (FM 11). Families, comments another, might not, 'understand that their Dad or the Mum has changed lately or over a period of time. They can still remember them a year or two years ago when they were living with them in the house' (FM 3).

These instances of empathy worked towards humanising people with dementia in residential care, helping create a sense of mutuality, so that care workers thought they too might respond, given the circumstances, in the same ways. As one suggests:

> If the resident is aggressive ... I suppose it's a measure of your own internal sort of reaction. If you really feel like this resident doesn't want this, it wouldn't be best for the resident, then it's probably better not to.
>
> (CW 1)

Certain behaviours were framed as logical, mutually explicable responses to care interactions, the social setting and the surrounding environment. Behaviours were viewed not just as expressions of unmet need, but reasonable reactions to environmental triggers. This suggests a shift away from simply viewing people with dementia as strange, and towards respecting them as persons who respond in human, social and thus mutually explicable ways.

### Creating professional distance in staff-resident interactions

At times care workers felt they needed to distance themselves from the individuals and emotional states of those they were caring for. This was as much for managing their own emotions, as to enable care to proceed. Bailey and colleagues (2015) argue that the ability of care workers to detach or distance themselves 'from the truth of the patient's situation' is required to keep a level of engagement intact. At times, they continue, care workers need to put aside certain feelings in order to fulfil their role. We observed a process by which care workers distanced themselves through physical (non-)presence, verbal exchange and communication and through managing their own feelings.

The most common distancing approach, one repeated by most care workers, involved backing off and physically removing oneself from a volatile situation. This was considered apt for dealing with aggression, but required one to delay the completion of a given task. Asked about dealing with aggression when attempting to provide care, one care worker's response was typical: 'I just maybe decide to leave that person for a day, maybe that resident is having a bad time. I will just maybe walk away and come back later' (CW 14). Thus, for most, putting aside the need to complete tasks to set a timeframe, was part of the daily routine, but could challenge their own perceptions of role performance. In such circumstances some might 'push' and pressure residents. As one care worker suggested: 'I have worked with some care staff that feel that they need to always meet the line and get them for a shower and make sure. And particularly if a resident's aggressive they feel that they must keep pushing' (CW 1).

Residents refusing the advances or help of care workers, was common, which one care worker felt should not be taken to 'heart': 'Let's take medication for example. People who don't want to take medication for whatever reason … Maybe they don't like you, maybe they don't like what you're wearing. There's a thousand things why they might say no' (CW 17). Critical was the ability to detach from the offence taken or sense of failure that could arise from residents refusing care. Most care workers accepted that a colleague might be better suited to a particular resident or task; switching care workers to suit the individual's mood or preference involved care workers accepting that they might not be best placed to engage with a resident: 'You're not going to go in there and upset them', states a care worker, 'there will normally be one person that they will relate to, [and] then that's what you draw on' (CW 21).

Communication was also a way to create a sense of distance. Most care workers warned against being over-familiar when communicating with residents. The use of nick names or terms such as 'nana', for example, were frowned upon (CW 2), with most preferring to use formal titles of address. Others suggested the need to 'just talk to them like anyone else', even if a situation might provoke feelings of sympathy and the sense of another's misfortune (CW 15). One care worker in particular stated in relation to interacting with a resident: 'She would be very angry with you, she'd call you names but you just get on with the job' (CW 18), indicating an ability to distance oneself from offence when required.

Another explained that while harsh words and potential aggression were experienced as 'infuriating', such feelings had to be put to one side in order to care (CW 9).

Care workers also felt they had to distance themselves from feelings of vulnerability that residents often expressed, particularly when needing assistance to shower. Aware that residents often felt embarrassed while naked, one care worker stated:

> As you can imagine it is extremely invasive having someone in there while you're very vulnerable, with no clothes on, so ... we chat about stuff to take peoples' minds off, you know that they're feeling vulnerable. We talk about family history, we talk about their feelings, we talk about the day, we talk about anything in general.
>
> (CW 17)

In this case distancing oneself from the resident's sense of vulnerability, enabled care workers to engage on a different level. In this way, task and relational care could be combined, as the following indicates:

> Q How would you shower someone who didn't want to be showered?
> A You wouldn't just drag them, you'd be spending the time trying to build some sort of trust with that resident. You'd have an excellent setup happening. You'd have everything possibly on hand that you may need. There would be a lot of soothing talk, emphasis on words like warm water, that sort of thing. And you'd be doing it as quickly as you could, the quicker the better.
>
> (CW 24)

As indicated the task is performed within a relational frame, and swiftly, so as not to prolong a potentially distressing situation.

Distance might also work another way. Advised never to challenge residents with dementia, care workers often detached from the reality of a given situation in order to engage with the resident. This might occur when someone wanted to return to their old home, or when someone was waiting for a visitor who had long since died. In such situations care workers went along with the person, aware that revealing the facts might cause distress. '[Y]ou have to go with them, you can't fight them', states a care worker, 'I mean you can't go against ... if they're looking for their Mum you say "Well yes, your Mum is coming later this afternoon" and try and divert, but go with them. You can't say "Well your Mum's dead"' (CW 3).

### *Adopting a problem-solving approach*

Empathic understanding balanced with different ways of creating distance enabled problem-based approaches to the puzzle of dementia care to be adopted.

The ability to stand back and assess the feelings underpinning particular behavioural responses or environmental factors triggering certain responses enabled facility managers and care workers to better reason on what might be causing someone to feel unhappy, distressed or anxious.

The final piece of seeing dementia care as a puzzle becomes problem-solving, which care workers expressed as a continuous process. 'It's problem-solving every day', states a care worker, 'to make these people's lives as best as they can' (CW 21). And, according to a facility manager, who cast the matter in different terms: 'we're continually evaluating strategies on how we manage residents' (FM 13).

Again, knowing the resident proved critical. For instance, someone who usually rises early and is not up could indicate an issue needing attention. '[Y]ou need to...know them individually, know what triggers them, what can make them upset, what can make them angry, how to reduce that behaviour and you only get to know that by getting to know the resident' claims a care worker (CW 21).

Such knowledge provides a basis for action. As a facility manager states: 'when residents with dementia do things that they don't normally do, we normally have a look at what might be going on ... sometimes there are a lot of patterns to residents' behaviour' (FM 13). '[We] know their behaviours', claims a care worker, 'changes to which might indicate an infection or that something else is wrong' (CW 20). By monitoring patterns of behaviour, such as when a resident usually gets up in the morning, care workers were ready to intervene if they noticed changes occurring; they communicated several options open to them, such as reporting their concerns to colleagues or supervisors, updating care plans and resident records, seeking medical assistance and speaking with the resident's friends or relatives.

Once detected, the cause of particular behaviours might, according to a facility manager be approached by,

> standing back and ... pulling together all of the evidence and what the reasons for the behaviour could be. Having a look to see if the resident is unwell or if they've got an infection. Then getting involvement of a multidisciplinary team approach ... doing assessments and having a look at what ... could be the reasons for the changes in the behaviour.
>
> (FM 6)

A range of explanations might be drawn on in such a process. This could involve, as mentioned above, medical reasoning. However, care workers and their managers could also draw on social and cultural explanations, gauged through knowing the resident:

> So with dementia care you need to know who is that person, what makes them tick, what did they like to do, what did they hate to do, what got up their nose, what aspects of their life 30–40 years ago are so embedded in

their understanding that we need to be aware of. So that if the man was an accountant and you sit down and start writing, he's going to want to join in and you are much better to give him a paper and some figures and a pen. And even though it's not making any sense, he will default to that behaviour … That's where he'll feel comfortable.

(FM 11)

Other social and cultural explanations for particular behavioural responses drawn from the evidence include men or women not wanting to be showered by the opposite sex, interpersonal dynamics between residents, cultural values linked to gender roles and preferred foods, and according to one senior manager (SM 9), residents feeling lonely or bored. These too could be solved through balancing empathy and distance.

The challenge was that the problems that arose and solutions developed were likely to change without notice. 'And what is frustrating for the staff', states a facility manager, 'is they develop a strategy that seems to work one day and then the next it doesn't, so they've got to go back to the drawing board and start again … they're always thinking about what can we do next?' (FM 12).

The process of 'trial and error' involved in daily dementia care, parallels the notion of care as 'practical tinkering' and 'attentive experimentation' (Mol *et al.* 2010), but might also be seen as working with multiple frames of dementia – medical, social, emotional and so on.

The ability of care workers to approach dementia care as a puzzle rests on the organisation's ability to create the right opportunities, and enable some level of flexibility and discretion. From a regulatory perspective this might be seen as 'variation within limits' (Gray and Silbey 2014), and crucially, permitting the inclusion of social and cultural experience into the equation. Through this strategy regulation shifts to the background, as a framework to guide, but not over-determine, care conduct, enabling a space for creativity and social experience.

## Discussion

Government regulation plays an important role in achieving policy objectives and instrumental goals such as safety and maintaining care standards. These are important aspects of regulatory control and oversight. Examining the ways care workers respond to regulation, interpret and adapt standardised controls to particular care settings and use regulation to moderate inter-personal interactions adds another frame to better understand dementia care. A distinction between hard and soft regulations is particularly useful, suggesting a middle-ground or interpretive space, which provides opportunities for the flexible implementation of regulation in residential care. As Heimer (2008, 2013) suggests, soft regulation helps organisation match regulation with the realities of everyday care. This is significant for a number of reasons. Standardised regulatory controls can be adapted to the dementia care setting and to individuals, leaving space for organisations and their staff to respond in nuanced ways. Further, by making compliance routine, such is the case with practices around food safety and manual handling, care workers can potentially attend to 'the important things' (CW 1), interacting with residents and adapting routines to suit individual needs.

The different ways organisations and care workers respond to regulation can both hinder and help dementia care. An examination of the everyday presents a complex picture of care worker conduct in light of competing demands. Significantly, care workers must manage their own emotions within an uncertain social environment at the same time as they are expected to connect emotionally with residents. Examining how this occurs in dementia care reveals that care workers are not powerless and simply controlled by regulation. They exercise agency, particularly in determining which rules need to be strictly followed and which can be enacted flexibly, and in strategising their conduct in response to multiple demands.

Care organisations and their workers can use rules and routines to manage the uncertainties of daily dementia care, as well as emotional connection. Routinised behaviours, reporting practices and overly prescriptive interpretations of guidance can prevent care workers from engaging with residents on a personal and emotional level. In this approach, regulatory rules and set tasks are prioritised so that meeting them comes to be seen as the chief goal of daily care, and emotional engagement becomes a secondary concern. This scenario arises primarily through time demands, which precipitate a focus on task and what is essential in terms of compliance, paperwork and the stresses associated with compliance monitoring.

On the other hand, regulation might be pushed to the background, as a framework that stipulates limits to practice and behaviour, but leaves space for creativity. One creative approach in particular – viewing dementia care as a puzzle – combines empathic understanding and distancing in a problem-based approach to dementia. While empathy was largely expressed by care workers and facility managers as knowing the individual, it also involved mutual understanding of emotional states, and recognising triggers in the care environment that might provoke certain behavioural responses. Creating distance between care workers and residents was used to avoid volatile situations, communicate effectively and help care workers manage their own feelings. Undergirded by 'knowing the person', distancing from the immediate feelings that certain interactions evoked, helped maintain personal connections on other levels with residents. Together, empathy and distancing facilitated a problem-based approach to daily dementia care, in what we have described as a puzzle approach towards dementia care. Seeing such care as a puzzle provides space for effective interventions in daily care to be devised.

The organisation and conduct of dementia care is a complex undertaking, involving multiple, often competing frames of reference. This discussion has shown how person-centred care, emotional work and engagement and regulation intersect in daily dementia care. Balancing multiple frames of reference is necessary in formal care settings, prompting in turn, the need for creative approaches.

One in particular – the puzzle approach to dementia and care – provides care workers with a useful framework for balancing and meeting the competing demands they encounter on a daily basis. It is also an effective approach to fostering positive staff-resident interactions plus managing the complex emotions involved.

# References

Armstrong, P., 2017, Balancing the tension in long-term residential care, *Ageing International*, 43(1): 74–90.

Australian Government, 2014, *The Australian Government Guide to Regulation*, Canberra, Australia: Department of the Prime Minister and Cabinet.

Australian Government Department of Health, 2016, *2015–16 Report on the Operation of the Aged Care Act 1997*, Canberra, Australia: Department of Health.

Australian National Audit Office, 2014, *Administering Regulation: Achieving the Right Balance*, Canberra, Australia: Australian Government.

Bailey, S., K. Scales, J. Lloyd, J. Schneider, R. Jones, 2015, The emotional labour of health-care assistants in inpatient dementia care, *Ageing & Society*, 35(2): 246–269.

Banerjee, A., P. Armstrong, T. Daly, H. Armstrong, S. Braedley, 2015, 'Careworkers don't have a voice': Epistemological violence in residential care for older people, *Journal of Aging Studies,* 33: 28–36.

Behuniak, S. M., 2010, Toward a political model of dementia: Power as compassionate care, *Journal of Aging Studies*, 24(4): 231–240.

Brooker, D., 2004, What is person-centred care for people with dementia? *Reviews in Clinical Gerontology*, 13(3): 215–222.

Brooker, D., 2005, Dementia Care mapping: A review of the research literature, *The Gerontologist*, 45(s1): 11–18.

Brooker, D., 2007, *Person-Centred Dementia Care: Making Services Better*, London: Jessica Kingsley.

Buse, C., J. Twigg, 2016, Materialising memories: Exploring the stories of people with dementia through dress, *Ageing & Society*, 36(6): 1115–1135.

Crichton, J., T. Koch, 2007, Living with dementia: Curating self-identity, *Dementia*, 6(3): 365–381.

Davis, D., 2004, Dementia: Sociological and philosophical constructions, *Social Science and Medicine*, 58(2): 369–378.

DeForge, R., P. van Wyk, J. Hall, A. Salmoni, 2011, Afraid to care; unable to care: A critical ethnography within a long-term care home, *Journal of Aging Studies,* 25(4): 415–426.

Fine, M., 2015, Cultures of care, in J. Twigg, W. Martin (eds), *Routledge Handbook of Cultural Gerontology,* pp. 269–276, Abingdon, UK: Routledge.

Freiberg, A., 2010, *Re-Stocking the Regulatory Tool-Kit*, Working Paper No. 15, June 2010, Israel: The Hebrew University.

Gray, G.C., S.S. Silbey, 2014, Governing inside the organization: Interpreting regulation and compliance, *American Journal of Sociology,* 120(1): 96–145.

Haines, F., 2011, *The Paradox of Regulation: What Regulation Can Achieve and What it Cannot*, Cheltenham, UK: Edward Elgar.

Heimer, C.A., 2008, Thinking about how to avoid thought: Deep norms, shallow rules, and the structure of attention, *Regulation and Governance*, 2(1): 30–47.

Heimer, C.A., 2013, Resilience in the middle: Contributions of regulated organizations to regulatory success, *The ANNALS of the American Academy of Political and Social Science*, 649(1): 139–156.

Herskovits, E., 1995, Struggling over subjectivity: Debates about the 'Self' and Alzheimer's Disease, *Medical Anthropology Quarterly*, 9(2): 146–164.

Hochschild, A.R., 1983, *The Managed Heart: Commercialization of Human Feeling*, Berkeley and Los Angeles, USA: University of California Press.

Hochschild, A.R., 2003, The culture of politics: Traditional, postmodern, cold-modern and warm-modern ideals of care, in A. Hochschild, *The Commercialization of Intimate Life: Notes from Home and Work*, Berkley, USA: University of California Press.

Hoggett, P., 2000, *Emotional Life and the Politics of Welfare*, Basingstoke, UK: Macmillan.

Hughes, J.C., 2006, Patterns of practice: A useful notion in medical ethics?, *Journal of Ethics in Mental Health*, 1(1): 1–5.

Hunter, P.V., T. Hadjistavropoulos, S. Kaasalainen, 2016, A qualitative study of nursing assistants, *Ageing and Society*, 36(6): 1211–1237.

Kitwood, T., 1997, *Dementia Reconsidered: The Person Comes First*, Buckingham, UK: Open University Press.

Kitwood, D., K. Bredin, 1992, Toward a theory of dementia care: Personhood and well-being, *Ageing and Society*, 12(3): 269–287.

KPMG, 2014, *Applicability of Consumer Directed Care Principles in Residential Aged Care Homes*, Final Report, Canberra, Australia: Department of Social Services.

Lopez, S.H., 2006, Emotional labour and organized emotional care: Conceptualizing nursing homes care work, *Work and Occupations*, 33(2): 133–160.

Mavromaras, K., G. Knight, G, L. Isherwood, A. Crettenden, J. Flavel, T. Karmel, M. Moskos, L. Smith, H. Walton, Z. Wei, 2017, *2016 National Aged Care Workforce Census and Survey – The Aged Care Workforce, 2016*, Canberra, Australia: Department of Health.

McCormack, B., 2003, A conceptual framework for person-centred practice with older people, *International Journal of Nursing Practice*, 9(3): 202–209.

McCormack, B., 2004, Person-centredness in gerontological nursing: An overview of the literature, *Journal of Clinical Nursing*, 13(s1): 31–38.

Menzies Lyth, I., 1988, *Containing Anxiety in Institutions: Selected Essays*, London: Free Association Books.

Mol, A., I. Moser, J. Pols (eds), 2010, *Care in Practice: On Tinkering in Clinics, Homes and Farms*, Bielefeld, Germany: Transcript Verlag.

Pols, J., 2004, *Good Care: Enacting a Complex Ideal in Long-Term Psychiatry*, PhD thesis, The Netherlands, Utrecht: Trimbos Institut.

Tronto, J., 1994, *Moral Boundaries: A Political Argument for an Ethic of Care*, New York: Routledge.

Venturato, L., W. Moyle, A. Steel, 2011, Exploring the gap between rhetoric and reality in dementia care in Australia: Could practice documents help bridge the great divide?, *Dementia: The International Journal of Social Research and Practice*, 12(2): 251–267.

# 11 Why 'person-centred' care is not enough

## A relational approach to dementia

*Gaynor Macdonald*

### Dementia as social challenge: a relational approach

The dementia space might seem an unlikely context in which to find a radical social movement. Dementia could be said to lie on the edges of social life. Those with diseases that produce cognitive degeneration are often isolated or stigmatised, assumed unable to participate; those who care for them find themselves marginalised; and those without direct experience are fearful, often discriminatory or in denial. Yet, as concern about attitudes towards, and care of, those with dementia mount in response to increasing incidence, fresh and challenging ideas are invigorating this space.

The term that people are using to explore new modalities of dementia care is relational care. To some, this is an extension of the well-established person-centred approach: it is about 'doing care better'. I argue that it is much more. It is not simply an approach to care: it is a new way of thinking about what it means 'to be'. This is what is radical about a relational approach.

Dementia is an important place to think about what it means 'to be'. It seems to challenge what people in the modern western world have been taught to believe about our humanness. Yet the dominant western cultural understandings are getting in the way of good care. I consider that relational care was the intention of Tom Kitwood in the 1990s, when he established the need for person-centred dementia care, but the way in which he defined personhood has allowed his intention to be derailed. Anthropology's debates on personhood and change have been central to my research over many years. When my husband was diagnosed with Alzheimer's in 2013, I could see an awkwardness in understandings of personhood in the dementia literature.

To understand ourselves as relational beings challenges the philosophical traditions of the western world, the idea that humanness is located within a rational, individualised entity – a human being as a separate, embodied person. As relational selves, rather than individuals, we understand ourselves as *constituted within relationship* – with other people, the non-human world of gods, animals, plants, with ideas and objects; all those 'things' with which we make connections. The quality of our lives depends on the quality of the relationships within which we are entangled at any point in our lives, and we do not exist outside of these.

Much has been written about the strengths of a person-centred approach to dementia care. It has become the major practice value in professional care today. But Kitwood's ideas also find themselves on rocky paths: ignored, misconstrued, watered down, reconfigured so as to be less confronting, and for a variety of reasons. Many people and institutions are forging ahead, with encouraging practices; others are resistant to change and its economic costs; and yet others glimpse the value of his approach, but do not quite understand its implications. I start by examining the person-centred approach to show why the thinking upon which it is conventionally based gets in the way of its effectiveness. What people who adopt this approach really desire will be better achieved by thinking about ourselves as relational beings rather than as individualised persons. This is more than a change of wording. A relational approach implies that good care, in any context, but perhaps especially in that of dementia, is a reflection of the *quality* of relatedness. This goes further than person-centred care because it cannot be conceptualised outside of the *relationship of connection* formed between carer(s) and those cared for. A relational-care model requires that we conceptualise ourselves as relational beings. I expand on this below but first I outline the dominant model of humanness in the western tradition, showing how this impacts on thinking about persons, and on dementia care.

## Persons as substance: the Cartesian influence

The 2001 *A Handbook of Dementia Care* was organised around different approaches to dementia, including: biomedical and clinical perspectives; psychological; sociological; philosophical and spiritual; and the perspectives of people with dementia, their families and their carers. There is nothing unusual about this list, although different approaches do not necessarily speak to each other well, and they do not get the same airing in public space. Had there been an anthropological section, perhaps cultural (including religious/spiritual) differences in thinking about humanness might have been more evident. But to the extent that these approaches are developed within a western tradition of knowledge and research, all are likely to assume a certain understanding of a human being.

How a relational approach to dementia care differs from the person-centred approach requires some understanding of the medical tradition within which dementia research takes place. Alzheimer's discovery, that dementia was a disease of the body, a neurological condition, meant dementia was amenable to biomedical intervention; a site of treatment, cure or avoidance. Neurological understandings of dementia emerged within a medical science that was founded on a definition of humanness developed in the seventeenth century by René Descartes (1996). His ideas remain influential in medicine. Descartes argued that people were not simply constituted by God. Rather, a human being, although made by God, becomes an autonomous subject in his own right, self-consciously able to act in the world of his own accord, able to shape that world. He was an individual, with an independent, tangible, material body as well as an intangible, immaterial mind. This subject is capable of reason and of ascertaining truth. Descartes demythologised the body, allowing it to be acted on upon, even reshaped. In the western tradition, human beings were henceforth disconnected from their complete dependence on, and control by, God.

Medical science adopted Descartes' reasoning that the subject of their study, the body, was like a machine, made up of material properties and subject to mechanical laws (Quesnell 2004). Knowledge could be acquired that meant disease or damage could be understood and interventions designed to rectify abnormalities. Research into the body and its workings has since transformed the quality of human life for countless people, as it will no doubt one day achieve in the context of dementia.

Descartes saw that mind could control body, and body could influence mind but mind was non-material and had no laws: it could not be studied in the same way. His model is known as Cartesian dualism: the mind:body split (Mehta 2011). This demythologising meant a redefining of humanness, from God's creation to an individualised substance (body) with an intangible mind. Earlier western philosophers had valued reason and rationality but Descartes made this the supreme characteristic, later reinforced by, for example, Kantian individualism. Not only medicine but also moral and social philosophy thereafter imagined human beings as rational, autonomous embodied individuals.

Dementia sits awkwardly in this body:mind space. Dementia is challenging not only because it eludes cure but because it so clearly has social and moral expressions that a biomedical approach cannot address. It is body:mind:social. Medicine's focus is research on brain pathology, or how drugs might alleviate 'challenge behaviours'. But *living with* dementia, for all involved, is a *social experience*, beyond the conventional domain of 'medicine'. This leads to what Mehta (2011) calls the 'paradigmatic error', the discordance between what contemporary medical professionals have to offer and what lay people expect from them (cf. Kleinman 2015).

The vulnerability produced by memory loss and disorientation changes what it means to live in the world. As the disease progresses, impacts on others are arguably more intense than they are for the person with the disease: carers – family members, friends, health workers, neighbours and others in daily contact. Interpersonal and social dimensions are left to allied health professionals (including, for example, nurses, psychologists, occupational therapists, professional care workers) and family members, people who (with the exception of some psychiatrists) do not have the status or resources of medical professionals, even though they are the ones who will see a person through the dementia experience. The medical paradigm of dementia as individualised body-substance with (incurable, barely treatable) brain pathology gets in the way of the need for greater social and economic investment into the experiences of dementia in a *social, relational context*. This is where the notion of person-centred care comes in – but it is not enough: the person of the patient is not the only person to consider.

## The limitations of 'person-centred' care

Through the twentieth century, medicine's somatic paradigm was exacerbating a lack of consideration of the social and psychic dimensions of dementia. Concern was mounting:

> Back in the early 1970s, at a time of rapid growth of high technology, reductionism, and bureaucracy in medicine, there had been rising anxiety that clinicians weren't treating patients as individuals whose lives and disorders had a richly human background and social context. ... physicians' narrow focus on diagnosis and treatment led them to miss or intentionally exclude the centrality of the patient's experience.
>
> (Kleinman 2015: 1376)

This was the context in which, in the 1990s, psychologist Tom Kitwood (1937–1998) sought to change the somatic ordering of dementia that had treated people as worthless, little more than the living dead. Person-centred care placed the onus on carers to treat a person with dementia as a person of value, stepping in where biomedicine could not go. Dementia was not simply a brain disease, it manifested in a progressive loss of personhood: care must therefore be person-centred, focused on what 'remained' of this person at any point. This was a game changer. It is now well-established that higher levels of challenging behaviour, distress or apathy can be expected to occur more commonly in care settings that are not person-centred, and the influence of person-centred care now extends into research and practice across different care contexts.

But what did Kitwood mean by the person? His most frequently cited definition is that personhood is 'a standing or status that is bestowed upon one human being, by others, in the context of relationship and social being. It implies recognition, respect and trust' (1997: 8). This is not a definition of humanness, of what 'being' means. Rather, personhood is the status given to a person, within a particular cultural context, *by others*. It is not about who one *is* but what value others *choose to bestow* (see Baldwin and Capstick 2007). Therein lies its contradiction. Not all people are bestowed standing or status of social value, as is evident in cases of racism, sexism or ageism. A person (usually) has autonomy and rights, but slaves and criminals are denied both, even if seen as human, and some women, children and elderly people are also denied these.

Is Kitwood suggesting that all people, regardless of standing or status, should be accorded 'recognition, respect and trust'? In which case, he is not talking about personhood but about being human, *regardless* of the status bestowed. Or is he saying that all carers of those with dementia must accord 'standing and status' to someone with dementia, regardless of the way in which they are recognised more widely? This not only puts pressure on a carer's own attitudes, prejudices and beliefs, but it does not recognise that it is a social order that confers status, not an individual. How does one deal with the politics and economics of status and stigma in the wider world, and then change one's cultural-social attitudes when entering a home or institution to care for someone with dementia, someone who may challenge one's conceptions of social value?

> *Gaynor*: Our (professional, trained) carer had been looking after my husband (mild to moderate Alzheimer's) all morning before bringing him to meet me so we could attend a work function together. He arrived unshaven and poorly dressed and I was embarrassed for both of us. When I asked her about it later, pointing out the importance to him of his dignity, and his dependence on us to maintain it, she responded that it didn't matter because he was old and he wouldn't know anyway.

Kitwood's inadequate definition confuses humanness (being) with person-hood (social status or standing). He appears to ignore how values differ in every society. Persons are not all equal. This becomes stark when those less socially-valued become dependent: older women experience more discrimination, as do those who are poor.

There is a lack of published work that has sought to critically assess and distil the theoretical, methodological and professional inroads forged by the concept of person-centred care (cf. Carr and Biggs, this volume). Four assumptions commonly emerge. One is that *personhood is a static attribute, it does not change over an adult's lifetime but can be lost with cognitive decline.* This runs counter to the lived experience of all people: the human lifecycle as well as personal histories. Change of all kinds is constant. This may include significant changes across a whole range of abilities, social, physical and mental. Any model of a personhood which can be 'lost' indicates a static and limiting conception of life. This links to the second idea, that *personhood depends on a capacity for rational social engagement*, an assumption that holds rationality as the totality of human engagement.

A third issue is that *persons are conflated with humans, and all have equal status and value.* This is contrary to the anthropological and philosophical distinction between humans as members of the human species (biological human-ity) and personhood, as a status given to some humans as well as non-humans and non-organic life. A person is culturally-constituted and socially-recognised, their moral status known through specific social norms (Mills 2011). Someone accorded status in one social context may not receive this in another situation. Fourth, person-centred care assumes *persons have status.* But who confers this status, and on what basis? This ignores the reality of discrimination and, in particular, that legal status is not accorded someone experiencing cognitive decline. A romanticised conflation of human and person is not helpful. It elides the value judgements that shape the dementia space: ageism, racism, sexism, poverty, class, place of residence, lack of education.

The prevalent idea of person-centred care, that we can learn about a person's life history as a way of attributing them status and treating them with more dignity, is a 'person-as-container' approach. If 'the person' is stuffed with values, experiences, memories, statuses and other paraphernalia thought significant by care professionals, it will slowly and inevitably be emptied as dementia progresses. The idea of personhood is only going to protect a person with dementia for as long as the container, as filled by others, is intact. So, despite Kitwood's efforts, the images of dementia as loss, disappearance and living death persist. This is limiting way of valuing the 'being' of someone who sits before you, at this moment of time.

There have been creative efforts to try to expand the model of personhood in the dementia space. Post (2016), for instance, critiquing the hyper-cognitive modern society, stresses that cognition does not embrace the totality of human experience. It does not account for emotions: passion, rage, grief, sadness, empathy; nor does it include the senses: touch, hearing, sight. But this still tends to leave the person-as-container model in place – it simply enriches the content of the container. The point, surely, must be that emotions and senses *allow all kinds of connection between people*, well beyond those associated with cognitive abilities.

Three web-based descriptions of person-centred care follow, obtained through a random Google search on 'person-centred care'. Only the first is dementia-specific. I use them to illustrate common limitations in representations of person-centred care. The first is a United States health information site, VeryWell (Heerema 2017). Note the use of 'remaining', implying emptying:

> Person-centered care also encourages and empowers the caregiver to understand the person with dementia as having personal beliefs, remaining abilities, life experiences and relationships that are important to them and contribute to who they are as a person.

A British site, written by professors of nursing, explains 'why getting to know the person behind the patient is the raison d'être of person-centred nursing care' (Draper and Tetley 2013).

> A person-centred approach to nursing focuses on the individual's personal needs, wants, desires and goals so that they become central to the care and nursing process. This can mean putting the person's needs, as they define them, above those identified as priorities by healthcare professionals. In the words of Bob Price, a nurse academic writing for the *Nursing Standard* in 2006, 'the term person-centred care is used…to indicate a strong interest in the patient's own experience of health, illness, injury or need. It infers that the nurse works with the person's definition of the situation, as well as that presented through a medical or other diagnosis'.

Another example is from the Australian College of Nursing (2014):

> The Australian College of Nursing (ACN) believes that the principle of person-centred care is a central tenet underpinning the delivery of nursing care and health care generally. Person-centred care means:

- treating each person as an individual;
- protecting a person's dignity;
- respecting a person's rights and preferences; and
- developing a therapeutic relationship between the care provider and care recipient which is built on mutual trust and understanding.

A nurse's ability to deliver person-centred care is determined by the attributes of the nurse; their nursing practice; and the care environment …

- Attributes of a nurse that enable her/him to deliver person-centred care include professional competence (the knowledge, skill, attitudes, values and judgements required); well-developed interpersonal skills; self-awareness; commitment to patient care; and strong professional values.
- Nursing practices that contribute to person-centred care include those that: acknowledge peoples' cultural and spiritual beliefs, preferences and rights; empower people to make informed decisions about their care; provide a sympathetic presence; and provide holistic care.
- Elements in a care environment that support person-centred care include; an appropriate staff skill mix; the presence of transformational leadership enabling the development of effective nursing teams, shared power, potential for innovation, supportive workplace culture and effective organizational systems); and the functionality and aesthetics of the built environment.

At a superficial level, there seems no reason to be critical of such statements. But in each example 'the person' is an individual, separate from the carer, whose autonomy must be respected, who can be understood as a unique individual, for whom care should be personalised; care can engage family and significant others. The carer is enjoined to learn as much as possible about the person being cared for. These are examples of a person-as-container approach. The container is filled with stories, experiences and names which constitute that person. In the first two, the carer is ignored, except as someone who is implicitly acting upon (occasionally with) another person. In the third example, there is appreciation that the carer is important to the care a person receives. Although this statement still wrestles with conventional thinking, it is striving to move beyond the person-as-container model to include the carer in a relationship. It refers to the nurse's own attributes and contains a key concept: self-awareness. It does not describe a relational approach but it hints at moving towards one.

The dominant model of personhood is thus a rational, self-aware, independently-functioning, autonomous and communicative individual, who inevitably loses personhood attributes when diagnosed with dementia. Personhood discourse might make for some better care practices but this model reinforces dementia as a form of death within life, the progressive and tragic unbecoming of life as 'a person' slowly diminishes before one's eyes (Macdonald 2018). Swinton (2012: 49ff) actually argues that descriptions and categorisations of dementia as loss and diminishment 'tend to result in a deep fragmentation and reduction of human persons'. In part, this is because the idea of 'the person' feeds into notions such as 'typical' and 'normal'. The language of personhood narrows understandings of a worthy life lived according to other, equally valid, criteria.

Although designed to counter the erasure of the person, 'recognising the person' is often turned into a 'technique' of care, a competency, undermining what it was meant to foster. It has become part of a carer toolkit, a mechanical task, something to record on a patient's file, ways to chat with them when they are agitated, reduced to occupying the time of the patient. It has become, to para-phrase Kleinman (2015), a kind of cultural-competency movement in which efforts to humanise care reduce complex lives to limiting stereotypes. The focus on the person as individualised container risks succumbing to glib deconstruc-tionism in lieu of responsible *engagement*. To chat to me about my dog, whose name is in your notes, can be annoying, even a disturbing expression of deper-sonalisation. 'I' am not the information contained in your file. Much of it is irrel-evant if you do not show me *in your attitude and body language* that you are interested in and wish to connect with me, *right now*.

It seems ironic that Kitwood (1997: 133) himself anticipated this:

> It is conceivable that most of the advances that have been made in recent years might be obliterated, and that the state of affairs in 2010 might be as bad as it was in 1970, except that it would be varnished by eloquent mission statements, and masked by fine buildings and glossy brochures.

Person-centred care has meant learning about the person/patient in Cartesian terms – the embodied person as a substance (container), full of (interesting) things (life-history), about which much can be known (questionnaires assist in knowing new patients), to be used in more sensitive care practice. This is a long way from Kitwood's intention: person-centred care was meant to *start with the carer*.

## The missing carer in person-centred care

Returning from Uganda after some years of teaching, where he would have encountered a very different understanding of humanness and persons, there seems no coincidence that Kitwood's first book was entitled, *What is Human?* (1970). He took up psychology, developing the person-centred approach to care. He was committed to the education of carers, having observed positive outcomes when care was of high quality. In 1992 he founded the Bradford Dementia Group. Its 'person-centred' philosophy was simple and expresses his intention: 'treat others in a way you yourself would like to be treated'. He wanted 'to provide students with an opportunity to explore and develop the feeling, emo-tional and intuitive parts *of themselves*, so as to enrich personal resources in their work and everyday life' (Fox 1999, emphasis added). The programmes he developed, the Person-Centred Approach and Dementia Care Mapping were unique. Dementia Care Mapping is an observational tool used to develop person-centred care practice and to gauge quality-of-life (Brooker 2005). Kitwood (1997: 4, emphasis added) described it as 'a serious attempt *to take the standpoint of the person with dementia,* using a combination of empathy and observational skill'. It records, for example, 'personal detractions', which are staff behaviours that have the potential to undermine the personhood of those with dementia; as well as 'positive events' that enhance personhood (Brooker 2005).

This understanding of person-centred care, *starting with the carer,* was inspirational. Kitwood assumed that, for people with dementia, wellbeing was a direct result of the quality of relationships they enjoyed with those around them: 'The *interdependency* of the quality of the care environment to the relative quality of life experienced by people with dementia is central to person-centered care practice' (Brooker 2005, emphasis added). It was essential to see personhood 'in relational terms': 'Even when cognitive impairment is very severe, an I-Thou form of meeting and relating is often possible. ... For presentness is the quality that underlies all true relationships, and every I-Thou meeting' (Kitwood 1997: 12, 119).

Kitwood's point here is clearly elaborated by Swinton (2012) in a Christian context. It is also well-developed by Hydén in *Entangled Narratives* (2017), one of most insightful studies yet on relationality in the context of dementia, for professionals as well as family, and whether or not of religious inclination. Hydén (2017:8) points out that, in Kitwood's view,

> an individual is not a person on his or her own, but only in relations to and with others. A relational view of personhood implies that others can support the personhood of individuals with dementia by supplying some of the cognitive and semiotic resources that the dementia lack. Other persons can even 'carry' the personhood of the other.

Thus, what is evident in Kitwood's approach, yet often missing from person-centred practice, is the importance he placed on interdependency, the relationship with the carer (cf. Brooker 2004, 2005). To move people away from medical models, depicting people as objects with no subjectivity or personhood, Kitwood identified psychological and social needs that were required for a good sense of wellbeing on the part of all. The six most fundamental were love, comfort, identity, occupation, inclusion and attachment. Steel (2016) points out that Kitwood intended reflection on what these mean *to us as carers,* not just what they mean to the person we care for. Kitwood intended *the person of the carer* to be the primary focus in person-centred care although, in many person-centred care vision statements, the carer is absent completely or side-lined.

This clearly begs the unvoiced question: who is the 'person' of the carer? A carer whose own values, meanings, understandings of life and death are inflexible and unreflected upon, does not make a good carer for someone with dementia. Many of what are euphemistically called 'challenging or compromised behaviours' are produced by inappropriate or ineffective approaches to a person with dementia, not what is going on in their brain. This is not a criticism – carers are rarely taught how to address such behaviours adequately. The 'sleep–wake cycle disturbance, screaming, crying, repeated calling out, and pacing' (Chenoweth *et al.* 2009) are understandably difficult for family members to manage, leading to carer distress and placement of people in residential care, where they may not fare better. Does that mean such symptoms cannot be dealt with? Sometimes, and in certain forms of dementia, this is the case. But many behaviours are exacerbated by the ways in which people are treated, leading to what Kitwood (1997) called malignant social psychology. There is clear evidence that agitation, for example, is significantly reduced with good care practice (Chenoweth *et al.* 2009).

> *Gaynor*: We visited family we had not seen for some time. Charlie was greeted appropriately but thereafter ignored. While I tried to ensure he felt included, others did not, and eventually he moved to sit by himself, making interaction harder but providing him relief from the chatter. A young person got him coffee and biscuits, which he appreciated. But I could see his agitation increasing so decided it was time to leave. As we left, one adult commented, 'Charlie seems very agitated'. Of course! He had just been ignored for the best part of two hours. Charlie was responding to a lack of interest, a social disengagement. This lack lay on a spectrum from awkward ignorance to bad manners. Had I been ignored in a similar way, I would have become just as agitated – although I might have responded differently.
>
> I recounted this story to a paid carer who, when faced with 'problem behaviour', would keep telling me I could do nothing because these were symptoms of dementia. I had meant the story to illustrate the difference between symptom and reaction but before I could finish, she was already at pains to reassure me that agitation was 'normal'. Dementia may have contributed to an inability to closely follow and engage in conversation, however the agitation was a reaction to a poor relational situation.

Research, and hence carer advice, into the relational dynamics that produce or exacerbate difficulties for carers is not prioritised. For example, inclusion and attachment are two of Kitwood's fundamental human needs. Steel (2016) points out that inclusion

> means that we want to be a part of something. If we feel left out then it makes us feel bad. People living with dementia may lose track of conversation easily, being mindful of their feelings of inclusion is important.

She continues, 'Our connections in life are also crucial to our feelings of well-being. Everyone wants to feel connected to something, or someone; often a combination of both'. It cannot, must not, be assumed that because someone has dementia these fundamental needs somehow disappear along with all the other 'loss' that is assumed.

> *Gaynor*: My husband is rarely agitated in social situations as I have learned how better to engage him, and am more demanding of others that they include him. When he decides to go out at night, he gets extremely annoyed to find a locked door and tries to violently open it. I have learnt how to pick an appropriate moment to distract him (so he will not turn his anger on me), to explain that it is night time, that we will go out in the morning. Perhaps he will return to bed, perhaps he needs a snack first. There is nothing 'irrational' about his thwarted desire to leave the house, or his anger at being 'locked in'. I would feel the same if I felt I needed to leave a place.

Kitwood argued that all behaviour had meaning. The behaviours deemed 'challenging' for carers had to be understood from the perspective of a person who may have difficulty communicating needs and desires in more conventional ways. It is as if they are speaking a different language through their words and actions. It is not that they are necessarily irrational, it is just they may not be able to communicate what is rational to them. The onus is on the carer to figure out what is being said. This can be difficult but is rarely impossible. The carer's self-reflexive attitude is crucial. It is they who must adjust, learn the new language, adjust again when the language changes. Good dementia care is not about 'a person' being acted upon. Relational care is about the quality of the relationship and empathy that the carer can establish with a person who is frequently – and understandably – experiencing extreme frustration, confusion and vulnerability.

## Relationality in the context of care

A relational understanding of humanness and social life is not new (see Emirbayer 1997). It argues that our experience of ourselves, of other humans, and the non-human world, is continually being constituted and reconstituted through *relationship*: 'all humans as such are essentially relational beings who by their very nature are always beings-in-relationships and are always in the world first and foremost as affective beings rather than thinking and contemplative ones' (Zigon 2014: 21). This is the basis for relational being – and thus for relational care. It starts with the assertion that none of us are monadic, isolable individuals: we are nothing without the relationships within which we are immersed.

Our relational capacity is immense. It takes in relations with the non-human world – to ancestors and gods, to the feared and inspiring places around us, to our pets, as well our commitments to ideas and social movements – we could go on and on. Zigon (2014) has called this attunement, being in tune with what is around us: objects, places, animals, events and imaginings. This 'assemblage' of entanglements makes us who we are, even as the assemblage is changing throughout our lives. We are always in an unfolding process of being, embedded 'within relationships and stories that shift over time and space' (Somers and Gibson 1994: 65, cited in Emirbayer 1997: 288).

Throughout life, our concern as humans is with expanding and maintaining relatedness, repairing relationships or working out how to disentangle from them. A relational situation may be affirming, have minimal or neutral impact, or be denying; there are situations that are, literally, soul-destroying while others are ecstatic. When relationships do not matter, there are no moral imperatives. When they do matter, morality is not something abstract, to be imposed on a relationship, but is a quality within the relationship itself. This applies as much to the person with dementia as any other. They need to be understood as embedded within a social world of carers, family, friends, health professionals, all of whom are shaping that person's experience of being, just as that person is shaping theirs. It is relatedness that constitutes any situation – an event, a gathering, a care context on a ward, including relations with the physical environment, the furniture, equipment, the view from the window.

It is because we are relational beings, not static containers, that we have the incredible human capacity to adjust, to deal with change, to confront trauma, confusion, despair and to be responsive. True, there are limits and extremes: suicide might be seen, on the one hand, as the act of someone unable to see the self-affirming value of any of the relationships within which she is engaged or, on the other hand, as the cry for recognition that brings us back into relationship even if only to punish or haunt.

Relational understandings are gaining traction in the context of dementia (cf. Greenwood *et al.* 2001; Moser 2011; Barnes *et al.* 2016; Dupois *et al.* 2016; Hydén 2017). It is arguably in this context that the challenge to change our thinking about who we are, and who we are *in relationship*, is pressing. Those diagnosed with dementia are dwelling in the world, but may have less ability to negotiate how to entangle or disentangle: they are dependent on affirming relational care to ensure they live well.

In contrast to the person-centred mission statements above, we should expect an equal focus on carers in organisations that explicitly embrace a relational approach. One example is the Irish Dementia Services Information and Development Centre (2014):

> The DSIDC subscribes to a holistic model of dementia that draws on research and clinical contributions made by both medicine, psychiatry and the social and behavioural sciences to better understand dementia. The professional activities of the DSIDC have developed from a practical knowledge-based perspective underpinned by the fundamental belief that people with dementia have a right to be treated with dignity and respect and that many of the so called problems associated with dementia can be minimised or resolved through creative thinking.

The DSIDC supports the relationship-centred care approach that recognises the importance of the interpersonal and intrapersonal relationships that exist between the person and others around them. The relationship forms the context within which caring occurs. The interconnectedness of the physical, spiritual, social and emotional aspects of wellbeing and illness is recognised and the practitioner responds to the experience of the person with dementia holistically. Exploring the meaning they attach to the experience of dementia provides insights and therapeutic avenues that are otherwise hidden. Their perspective on their world and what is happening to them is made explicit through the nurturing of positive relationships. It is the understanding of this experience that is key to promoting the wellbeing of the person with dementia.

A relational approach is also evident in provider Arcare's 2014 promotional video, *It Takes a Community.*

It is the carer who must seek forms of engagement that will hold a person in connection. Some carers intuitively 'get this', and want to; others do not or are ill-equipped to do so. Relationships are not techniques of interaction, and a relational approach is more than a strategy to include in a curriculum for health professionals. A relational approach means that everyone takes responsibility for the way they hold any other person in connection, regardless of the social status conferred on them – manager, cleaner, patient, nurse, daughter, spouse, neighbour – in an understanding of our mutual dependencies and the impact each of us has on those others in every situation in which we find ourselves.

A student of an online dementia unit was troubled about whether or not one could tell 'a lie' to someone with dementia. From a relational perspective, morality is not about 'judging, evaluating, and enacting the good or right, but instead to be about the making, remaking, and maintenance of relationships' (Zigon 2014: 20–21). What will make someone comfortable, reassured, held in connection is more important than abstract morality. Radical changes may have to take place in a carer's personal moral universe. They may need to shed taken-for-granted values and assumptions in order to understand how to live relationally. Some manage, a great many do not. The issue is that carers are not being taught how to make these adjustments: societies that focus on individuality and persons-as-containers rarely prepare them.

Dementia is not loss of personhood. As relational beings we cannot be contained or divided, we cannot be 'lost'. Relationality is not an attribute or skill, nor even a mode of relating. It is a way of being: 'To be and to be in relation becomes identical' (Zizioulas 1985: 89). But we can become isolated when others withdraw from relationship, when they refuse or are unable to be in relationship. This is tantamount to social death. For those with dementia (in fact, all of us) it creates what Kitwood called 'malignant psychology' (see Smith 2014 for a confronting list of attitudes that create the toxicity that is malignant care).

The person with dementia is changing, but they may lack awareness of these changes. The onus on those around them is to be aware for them and to change what being in relationship with that person means. Moser (2011) demonstrates how holding someone with dementia in connection means becoming less dependent on verbal communication, developing a broader repertoire of communicative strategies – touch, visual stimulation such as direct eye contact and pictures, sounds that soothe (voice tone, music), sight – and watching for move-ments or expressions that might indicate distress or pain. Infants are held in con-nection in this way: one learns to read and respond to signals such as facial expressions and different kinds of crying that signal hunger or distress. To hold a person with dementia in relationship requires this attention to detail – but it does not necessarily require certain types of knowledge.

> *Gaynor*: Nayana is wonderfully gregarious. When she met my husband, she chatted to him as she walked along the road beside him, engaging him all the time. I could tell he really hadn't a clue what she was talking about, and it didn't matter – to either of them. He smiled, nodded and agreed, laughed when she did. He was enjoying himself, responding to her evident interest in engaging with him, her body language, her animation. She knew nothing about him – not where he had grown up, if he had siblings, if he liked dogs, what he did for a living – and she wouldn't have learnt them anyway – he would have looked to me to 'remember' for him had she asked. But she had this amazing ability to draw him out. This was a *relationship*, not someone acting on what they thought they knew about 'a person'.

Engagement has limits: dementia will eventually impede connection as someone draws close to death. But a relational approach allows people to be held in connection a great deal longer because it recognises that *living* is not about the state of our bodies/minds, it is about being in relationship. The focus in dementia research should be on how each one of us learns to hold another person in con-nection, even as they change, as they become more vulnerable, more dependent, and how we adjust to their changing ability to connect.

## Vulnerability in human experience

Our relationships and our interdependencies are the key to our wellbeing, and all the more so in any situation of vulnerability. Vulnerability is not a deficit: it is part of our being. We find ourselves (if we are honest) in many such situations, throughout even the most stable and healthy of lives, but childhood and old age are the most demanding of those interdependencies. Butler (2015: 123ff.) argues that vulnerability is a condition of interdependency: it engenders alliances and shapes social institutions and infrastructures. While it challenges our very sur-vival, it also forges relationships (Das 2010), not only between people but between them and the nonhuman world.

There should not be one social value for workers, tax-payers or the self-funded, and another for those defined as a 'drain on the public purse': neoliberal capitalist economies create these value inequities. We need to resist the value and meaning of our lives being reduced to economics. Life is about relatedness, the quality of the connections we are able to maintain. We live well or not according to whether we are able to make positive affirming connections with others and they with us. This applies as much in a workplace or shopping centre as it does in a care facility or private home. Every encounter is an opportunity to hold another in connection or treat them as inconsequential. Anyone who has worked behind a counter knows the difference. So, too, do those with dementia.

To the extent that we do not connect well with those with dementia, we will them to a social death (cf. Branelly 2011). Connection is the core of relational being: death is its opposite. Death as disconnection is always primarily about the severing of *social* connection, of relationship. A healthy body in a state of social death is truly tragic. Only when a person's body no longer allows for social connection, as in advanced dementia, or in severe and unbearable pain, is that person really close to death.

Butler (2009) saw that people whose lives are regarded as of little value, who are even already in the midst of death, barely elicit pity or grief because they are not recognised as living. In asking the question, what is a life? she was not asking a doctor to determine whether a person has passed from life to death, but which lives are liveable. How are some, but not all, lives constituted as liveable and by whom – through which cultural ideas and forms of power? If a person with dementia is considered as in the first stages of death rather than the last stages of life, their life is of little consequence. While all life is precarious, this precariousness can be adjusted for in the decisions made about economic distribution, access to quality health and care and so on. Precarity is a 'politically induced condition in which certain populations suffer from failing social and economic networks of support and become differentially exposed to injury, violence, and death' (Butler 2015: 27). When political and economic decisions do not treat lives of equal value, they maximise precariousness. Dementia is an example of politically and culturally-induced precarity.

To argue that the only life worth living is the normalised, healthy and wealthy one is cultural violence. The stigma and fear, and even the enormous energy spent looking for the cure demonstrate that understandings and treatments are not neutral. Those with dementia and their carers find themselves in a different world, expected to live away from those who cannot cope with its 'demands'. It is hardly surprising that nursing home care is recommended; that geriatricians have low status within the medical profession; and that care staff are poorly paid.

Fear of dementia makes sense in the context of disconnection: it threatens disconnection before 'one's time'. People with dementia most often want to remain within their homes, among neighbours, family and friends, but the economic, social and educational resources to enable this are not forthcoming because this is a competitive not a relational society. Disconnection looms in absence of a guarantee of relational care: being sent to a nursing home regardless of one's wishes, where busy staff do not know you; being dependent in a society that disdains vulnerability. We fear the demeaning of our life more than we fear our mortality. This is normative violence (Butler 2004, 2009): the leaving of a vulnerable person to erasure and exclusion, exposed to physical and emotional harm. These forms of disconnection do not allow for a liveable life.

There are people who shy aware from the idea that we are vulnerable. On the contrary, we should foreground it as an integral experience of life, one we move in and out of in various ways, for various reasons, but is an ever-present aspect of any life. It is a part of being human, not a weakness or deficit. To recognise this is to free ourselves to care and to be cared for, and to know that care is what 'being' is about.

Kittay (2002) has shown how personhood is bound into cultural ideas, in particular liberal notions grounded in masculinist (white, independent, adult males) ideas about the normal human capacity for rationality and self-sufficiency. A person with dementia is not only abnormal from a biomedical perspective, but always also an abnormal 'person'. It is in this concept of the normal that medical ideas mesh with economic and social values in debilitating ways. A normal life at life's end means 'successful ageing', a term that assumes healthy, active and financially-independent lifestyles for those over 65 years of age (cf. Timonen 2016). This rejects the vast majority of ageing persons. By default they become the negative. The abnormal legitimises intervention, control, stigma and fear, reinforcing the normal as that which is valued, recognised, acceptable and included. As Butler (2004) argues, life is not made liveable for those who sit outside powerful social norms. They become wasted lives (Bauman 2004), social outcasts, a drain on the public purse, prone to abuse.

Normative conceptions have to be challenged (cf. Butler 1990, 2004) to make way for the vast majority of us, including those ageing with dementia, who live with vulnerability, including physical, cognitive, emotional, social and economic ups and downs – in other words, the vicissitudes of a normal human life. People whose lives 'deviate' from the norm – whether in terms of education, prosperity, gender, disability, ethnicity or age – live on the vast spectrum of human variability and diversity. Likewise, models of personhood that downplay irrationality, vulnerability, stress and the constant need for adaptability, end up stigmatising. Normal and perfect have become forms of cultural violence and social control.

## Holding people with dementia in connection

Most of us know when we are being held in connection. We work at building and maintaining connectedness, especially within families where this can be trying, or with colleagues at work. There are plenty of people we encounter for whom there is no connection (but even momentary connections with passers-by can be affirming) and there are others in which there is evident disconnect. Relational being means we can be subject to significant violence when people around us do not hold us in connection, when they refuse to care. This is dementia's challenge: the onus is on the carer to learn new ways of connecting, for as long as is possible. Not to maintain connection is to consign a person to social death (cf. Moser 2011: 713–715).

A relational approach does not deny the reality and objectivity of dementia as a biomedical condition, nor the desirability of a cure, but demonstrates a different way of *acting upon life*, and shaping ways of living and dying with dementia. It is explicitly about establishing and maintaining connection, on the understanding that *social connectedness* is fundamental to life. Relational care is a commitment to counteract or at least postpone the processes of disconnection that characterise dementia for as long the body allows for this. Drugs are welcome when they facilitate this.

To produce a 'dementia-friendly' society, a rethinking about what it means 'to be' in positive and affirming relationships is required. Person-centred care will only assist if all persons are understood as relational beings. Far more research is required on appropriate or useful responses to situations that dementia carers can learn (cf. Hydén 2017).

> It wasn't the dementia literature but a comment from a friend who had been through this experience: 'you have to roll with the punches'. He helped me understand that it was I who had to change in order to hold my husband in connection. I am often told how fortunate I am that Charlie is a calm, gentle person, easy to look after. Nonsense: he exhibits all the problems in the dementia textbook! But I have learnt to calm, reassure and engage him. I watch his reaction at people unprepared or unskilled to make connection with him. He responds to this denial aggressively. And I watch those who seem intuitively to know how to connect, and see him relax and laugh. There are extreme behaviours, for which our doctors provide medication to assist, and there are always new challenges.

A major push is coming from psychology. Clarke and Wolverson's (2016: 216) positive psychology approach to dementia also moves well beyond limited personhood approaches, to a relational view. They point out that

> a relational view of dementia cannot focus on the needs of any one individual or group of individuals but rather must address the needs of all those involved in supporting people with dementia, whether in an unpaid or paid capacity.

They, too, assert that the value that must be developed must be in society as a whole, is to create a more enriched environment for all (cf. Nolan *et al.* 2006). To be more inclusive of those with dementia, inclusivity and awareness of our relationality needs to be at the forefront of social experience, whether or not we have dementia.

Those with dementia require more than 'person-centred care': they need to know they live in a social world in which they will be held in connection, because that is what *being* is. This does not mean that people with dementia can always be held in connection. When they cannot, they have entered death, and palliative care takes over. Death comes when our body prevents us from being held in relationship, or when there is no one committed enough to ensure our connectedness. This is true of any relationship: to the extent that it is not held in connection, it dies. People move on, move away. Life does dole out the harshness of separation and alienation, which is why separation is deliberately used as punishment. This includes being deliberately ignored, being sent 'to your room', imprisonment and solitary confinement (often ineffective because it cannot be restorative).

We will all die, the ultimate disconnection. This is significantly ameliorated for those who believe in an afterlife, especially one in which they will be reunited: for these people, connection and reconnection remains strong. But disconnection is also the experience of too many who are not facing death but financial hardship, social stigma, disabling physical conditions – and dementia. Our social circumstances as well as our bodies can and do impede our capacity to be *in relation*. The extent to which this induces the suffering of disconnection depends on how caring our society is. Even the person with dementia does not want, and should not have, to live or die alone.

It is no less than a revolution that is needed. We will only change attitudes to dementia if we are committed to changing a society that stigmatises and disconnects by first, defining people as individuals; then treating a large percentage of these as abnormal, as people of deficit; and that is not committed, socially or economically, to holding people in relationship. Caring is always a relational concept, whether we are caring for children, sick people, our gardens, animals or a climate. When we use 'care' to describe particular behaviours, attitudes or relations, we make assumptions about the carer and the cared for: the act of caring is often associated with looking after dependents. A relational approach insists that many other relationships between people, such as manager, supervisor, friend, colleague, should be understood in terms of a responsibility to care. Awareness of ourselves as relational beings means we have to take responsibility for the impact we have on others – the choice is care or denial, connection or disconnection and, ultimately, life or death.

Change will not result from tinkering with policies but from people willing to change themselves. We can start with our own commitment to hold others in connection. There are two core questions: how can I make this person's life liveable by improving the way I hold him or her in connection – which is always first a question of relationship, not programmes or activities; and how do we challenge the situations in which we find ourselves such that others will understand these in relational terms. These are questions that need to be asked of every politician, bureaucrat and medical and health professional in the dementia space. They have the power and resources: they need the moral challenge.

Dementia is an important lens through which to understand the necessity for a social movement of this kind. If we can appreciate what it means to relate to, to hold in connection, even one person with dementia, we will have changed our own thinking about what it means to be in relationship with every other person. Dementia disturbs, not because it is a tragic way to end a life but because it sheds light on the meanings we give to life, relatedness and death – and finds them wanting (Macdonald 2018). We can use the challenges of relatedness we encounter in living with dementia as one lens through which to reimagine life as relational. A caring society is possible but it will involve ontological, moral and economic shifts that sometimes seem more illusory than the cure for dementia.

# References

Arcare, 2014, *It Takes a Community*, set at Arcare Helensvale, Queensland, Australia, Fire Films, www.youtube.com/watch?v=IUJWFWXz-wY [Accessed 08 February 2018].

Australian College of Nursing, 2014, Position statement on person-centred care, *Key statement*, November 2014, www.acn.edu.au/sites/default/files/advocacy/submissions/PS_Person-centered_Care_C2.pdf [Accessed 02 February 2018].

Baldwin, C., A. Capstick (eds), 2007, *Tom Kitwood on Dementia: A Reader and Critical Commentary*, Berkshire, UK: Open University Press, McGraw-Hill Education.

Barnes, M., F. Henwood, N. Smith, 2016, Information and care: A relational approach, *Dementia*, 15(4): 510–525.

Bauman, Z., 2004, *Europe: An Unfinished Adventure*, Cambridge, UK: Polity.

Branelly, T., 2011, Sustaining citizenship: People with dementia and the phenomenon of social death, *Nursing Ethics*, 18(5): 662–671.

Brooker, D., 2004, What is person centred care for people with dementia?, *Reviews in Clinical Gerontology*, 13(3): 215–222.

Brooker, D., 2005, Dementia care mapping: A review of the research literature, *The Gerontologist*, 45(1): 11–18.

Butler, J., 1990, *Gender Trouble*, New York: Routledge.

Butler, J., 2004, *Precarious Life*, London: Verso Books.

Butler, J., 2009, Performativity, precarity and sexual politics, AIBR, *Revista de Antropología Iberoamericana*, 4(3): i–xiii.

Butler, J., 2015, *Notes Toward a Performative Theory of Assembly*, Cambridge, USA: Harvard University Press.

Cantley, C., (ed.), 2001, *A Handbook of Dementia Care*, Buckingham, USA: Open University Press.

Chenoweth, L., M.T. King, Y. Jeon, H. Brodaty, J. Stein-Parbury, R. Norman, M. Haas, G. Luscombe, 2009, Caring for aged dementia care resident study (CADRES) of person-centred care, dementia-care mapping, and usual care in dementia: A cluster-randomised trial, *Lancet Neurology*, 8: 317–325.

Clark, C., E. Wolverston (eds), 2016, *Positive Psychology Approaches to Dementia*, London: Jessica Kingsley.

Das, Veena. 2010, Sexuality, vulnerability and the oddness of the human: Lessons from the Mahabharata. *Borderlands*, 9(3): 1–17.

Descartes, R., 1996, *Meditations on First Philosophy*, translated by John Cottingham, first published 1641 in Latin, Cambridge, UK: Cambridge University Press.

Draper, J., J. Tetley, 2013, The importance of person-centred approaches to nursing care, *Open Learn*, 15 March 2013, www.open.edu/openlearn/body-mind/health/nursing/the-importance-person-centred-approaches-nursing-care [Accessed 21 January 2018].

Dupois, S., C. MaAiney, D. Fortune, J. Ploeg, L. de Witt, 2016, Theoretical foundations guiding culture change: The work of the partnerships in dementia care alliance, *Dementia*, 15(1): 85–105.

Emirbayer, M., 1997, Manifesto for a relational sociology, *American Journal of Sociology*, 103(2): 281–317.

Fox, L., 1999, Obituary: Professor Thomas Kitwood. *Independent: Culture*, 6 January 1999, www.independent.co.uk/arts-entertainment/obituary-professor-thomas-kitwood-1045269.html [Accessed 21 January 2018].

Greenwood, D., D. Loewenthal, T. Rose, 2001, A relational approach to providing care for a person suffering from dementia, *Journal of Advanced Nursing*, 36(4): 583–590.

Heerema, E., 2017, Thomas Kitwood's person-centered care for dementia, *VeryWell: Alzheimer's Disease and dementia information for caregivers*, 24 May 2017, www.verywell.com/what-is-person-centered-care-in-dementia-97737 [Accessed 23 January 2018].

Hydén, L., 2017, *Entangled Narratives: Collaborative Storytelling and the Re-Imagining of Dementia*, Oxford, UK: Oxford University Press.

Irish Dementia Services Information and Development Centre., 2014, *Relationship Centred Approach to Care,* http://dementia.ie/about-us/relationship-centred-approach-to-care [Accessed 02 February 2018].

Kittay, E.F., 2002, When caring is just and justice is caring: Justice and mental retardation, in E.F. Kittay, E.K. Feder (eds), *The Subject of Care: Feminist Perspectives on Dependency*, pp. 256–276, Oxford, UK: Rowman and Littlefield.

Kitwood T., 1970, *What is Human?*, Westmont, USA: Inter-Varsity Press.

Kitwood T., 1997, The experience of dementia, *Aging and Mental Health*, 1: 13–22.

Kleinman, A., 2015, From illness as culture to caregiving as moral experience, *New England Journal of Medicine*, 368(15): 1376–1377.

Quesnell, W.R., 2004, Prevent disease by thinking differently than experts, *The Cartesian Model of Health Care Forum*, http://forum.wholeapproach.com/topic/ the-cartesian-model-of-health care.

Macdonald, G., 2018, Death in life or life in death?: Dementia's ontological challenge, *Death Studies*, 42(5): 290–297.

Mehta, N., 2011, Mind-body dualism: A critique from a health perspective, *Mens Sana Monographs*, 9(1): 202–209.

Mills, C.W., 2011, The political economy of personhood, *On the Human* blog, http://onthehuman.org/ 2011/04/political-economy-of-personhood/#n2.

Moser, I., 2011. Dementia and the limits to life: Anthropological sensibilities, STS inferences, and possibilities for action in care, *Science, Technology and Human Values*, 36(5): 704–722.

Nolan, M.R., J. Brown, S. Davies, J. Nolan, J. Keady, 2006, The senses framework: Improving care for older people through a relationship-centred approach, *Getting Research into Practice (GRiP) Report No 2.*, Sheffield, UK: University of Sheffield.

Post, S.G., 2016, 'Is grandma still there?': A pastoral and ethical reflection on the soul and continuing self-identity in deeply forgetful people, *Journal of Pastoral Care & Counselling: Advancing Theory and Professional Practice through Scholarly and Reflective Publications*, 70(2): 148–153.

Steel, T., 2016, Dementia training: Tom Kitwood's flower of emotional needs, *Search Care Jobs* blog, 9 February 2016, www.searchcarejobs.com/blog/dementia-training-tom-kitwoods-flower-emotional-needs [Accessed 21 January 2018].

Smith, P., 2014, Dementia care: The toxic nature of malignant care, *Dementia Care Expert, Quality Compliance Systems,* www.qcs.co.uk/dementia-care-toxic-nature-malignant-care/ [Accessed 10 February 2018].

Swinton, J., 2012, *Dementia: Living in the Memories of God*, Cambridge, UK: Eerdmans Publishing.

Timonen, V., 2016, *Beyond Successful and Active Ageing: A Theory of Model Ageing*, Bristol, UK: Policy Press.

Zigon, J., 2014, Attunement and fidelity: Two ontological conditions for morally being-in-the-world, *Ethos*, 42(1): 16–30.

Zizioulas, J., 1985, *Being as Communion: Studies in Personhood and the Church*, Crestwood, USA: St. Vladimir's Seminary Press.

# Index

Page numbers in **bold** denote tables.

Milton Keynes UK
Ingram Content Group UK Ltd.
UKHW040102071024
449327UK00019B/751